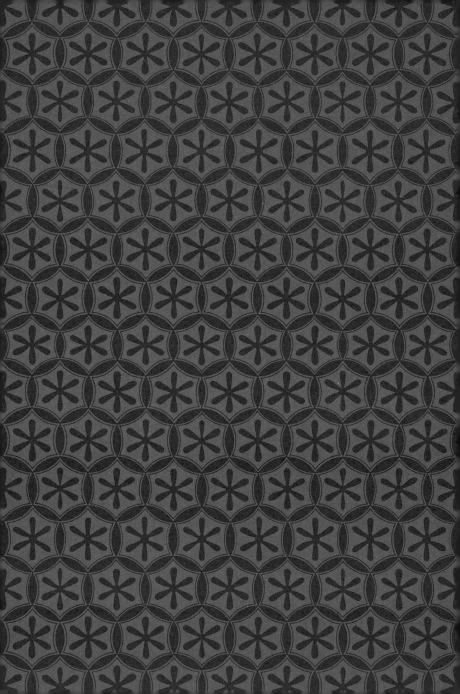

the art of manifesting

HQ

An imprint of HarperCollinsPublishers Ltd.
1 London Bridge Street
London SE1 9GF

www.harpercollins.co.uk

HarperCollinsPublishers
1st Floor, Watermarque Building
Ringsend Road
Dublin 4, Ireland

1
First published in Great Britain by
HQ, an imprint of HarperCollinsPublishers Ltd. 2022

Copyright © Carolyn Boyes

Carolyn Boyes asserts the moral right to be
identified as the author of this work

A catalogue record for this book is
available from the British Library
ISBN: 978-0-00-852306-0
Printed and bound in Latvia by PNB

Book Design: Steve Wells

All rights reserved. No part of this publication maybe reproduced, stored in a
retrieval system, or transmitted, in any form or by any means, elecronic, mechanical,
photocopying, recording or otherwise, without the prior permission of the publishers.

This book is sold subject to the condition that it shall not, by way of trade or otherwise,
be lent, re-sold, hired out or otherwise circulated without the publisher's prior consent
in any form of binding or cover other than that in which it is published and without a
similar condition including this condition being imposed on the subsequent purchaser.

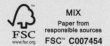

MIX
Paper from
responsible sources
FSC™ C007454

Our policy is to use papers that are natural, renewable and recyclable products and
made from wood grown in sustainable forests. The logging and manufacturing processes
conform to the legal environmental regulations of the country of origin.

Carolyn Boyes

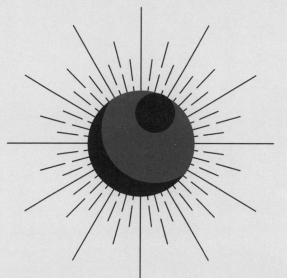

the art of manifesting

An imprint of HarperCollinsPublishers Ltd.

CONTENTS

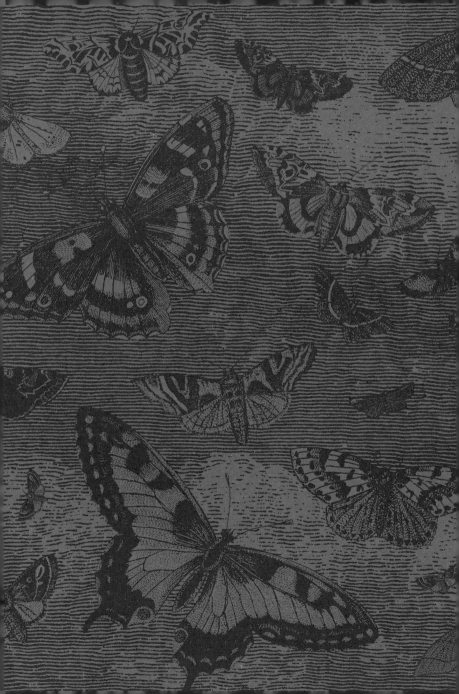

INTRODUCTION

D o you have dreams you've put off for way too long? Do you hunger for change in your life? But has the time never seemed right?

I know how it feels. Before I first discovered manifesting more than twenty years ago, I wanted big changes in my life. I had moved to another country and I knew what I was doing wasn't right for me, but I had no idea what to do next. I wanted a new job, a new relationship and to get my finances in order but I couldn't see what I could do to change things. I started to take courses and read widely about different traditions and philosophies. One wonderful teacher taught me a basic manifesting method and I wrote down my first ever intentional manifests.

After a while, I forgot about what I had written down, but nevertheless I started to take real steps to change my life. Eighteen months later, I was living back in my home country, in the apartment I had visualised, with new qualifications, a new job, and a new relationship. The changes I had imagined happening had all come true. I even had the exact amount of money in my bank account I had written down a year and a half previously.

Since I first learnt to manifest, I have studied many different spiritual and psychological disciplines. I have learned much more about the spiritual laws of the universe which help us to manifest, as well as how we can block manifesting from happening.

Manifesting is not a new idea. It has been tried and tested by the wisest people over thousands of years of human history. By creating a powerful picture in your mind of what you want and learning how to infuse it with intention, feeling and desire, you can learn how to create happiness in your life by the real results you manifest in the physical world.

Life is a journey and as you travel from birth to death a series of doors open for you. For many of us, we stumble through doors by accident without thinking much about our choices. When you intentionally manifest, it's different. You choose which doors you are going to open.

In the *The Art of Manifesting*, I will teach you how to change your life in a real and practical way by guiding you through a method which you will be able to use every day. My intention is to inspire you to think about the life you want to build and then discover how to build it.

Over the next eight chapters, you will discover the secrets of successful manifesting: the art of deliberately producing change in your world by harnessing the power of the universe to bring what you desire into existence.

Manifesting will allow you to become the person you were always meant to be with the life you were meant to live. It will give you true power over the course of your life and allow you to be the captain of your destiny.

If you have never dared to dream, it's time right now to plan and pursue a new future. If you already have dreams for a life not yet realised, it's time to start to activate them.

Be inspired by the infinite possibilities open to you right now and start your journey of manifesting today.

'You can't go back and change the beginning but you can start where you are and change the ending.'

C. S. Lewis

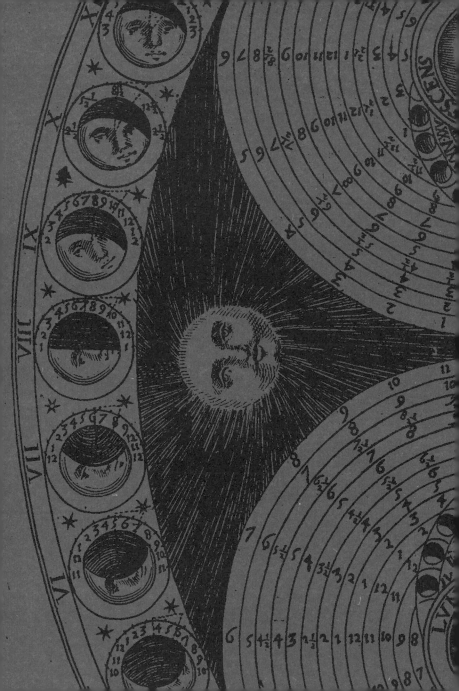

CHAPTER ONE

AWAKEN *to*
YOUR
POWER

'Happiness is your nature. It is not wrong to desire it. What is wrong is seeking it outside when it is inside.'

Ramana Maharshi

One day, Roshana was sitting in a café, drinking a cup of rapidly cooling coffee and feeling unhappy with her life. She had money worries, she constantly argued with her partner, she hated her job as an accountant, but she didn't know how to get out of the trap she had fallen into in her life. As she sat there staring at the coffee, she wondered, 'Is this the best I can hope for?' She sighed, 'I guess that's how it's always going to be. It's too difficult to change.'

Lots of us are like Roshana.

Do you ever feel unhappy? Anxious? Stressed? Sad? Hurt?

You would probably reply, 'Of course. Doesn't everyone?'

How about this?

Have you ever been broke, or lost your job? Did you have an unhappy childhood? Have you suffered illness or abuse? Have you ever felt you weren't in control of what is happening to you? Do you feel you can't change your future?

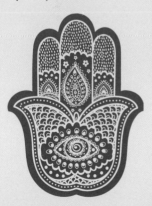

So many of us look at the world and don't know how to find our way to a better life. We think that we are subject to the forces of a hard world which is determined to cause us pain. Sometimes we think that if we had more power over our lives, things would change, but we go seeking power in the wrong places: in money, possessions or status. Then of course we still don't find the happiness we are looking for.

Life isn't supposed to be a series of negative emotions and constant suffering. Undoubtedly our experiences early in life cause us to think in a particular way. They lead us to have certain expectations about the life we will have. But they are not an inevitable signpost to our future.

There is an answer.

Over thousands of years, many secret groups have developed techniques to help people gain mastery over their personal lives through tapping into the power of thought and imagination. Until recently these techniques were seen as magical, occult or reserved for small groups of faith. These groups have been spread all over the world, but the techniques are always the same.

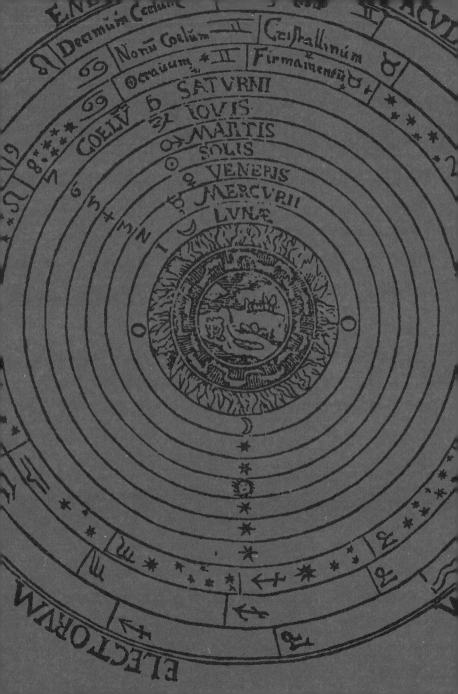

Things can change.

When you read about the lives of so many great historical figures, they have often been beset by horrific challenges from a young age, but these hard early experiences did not block them from also manifesting amazing accomplishments later in life.

Look at figures like Charles Dickens who experienced childhood poverty or Charlie Chaplin who was forced to live in an orphanage when young. Ludwig van Beethoven suffered from profound deafness. Nelson Mandela was imprisoned before he led a country. Those great figures from the past, managed to overcome these expectations and change their thoughts, feelings and experiences. It is the choices they made *despite* what they had been through which determined their destinies.

You don't have to accept that your past is your future.

Your life is your own.

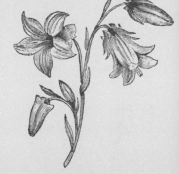

It doesn't matter who you are or what your current circumstances. Your hopes and dreams weigh the same as anyone else's and you deserve to bring them into being.

There is no one in the whole world exactly like you. You are an amazing, incredible person. You are meant to live an incredible life in this world. You were born to be happy and healthy and full of love. You were born to live in a world where love spreads to others through you.

The measure of success in your life is not the amount of material things you have or the awards and status you have achieved but your level of happiness. If you are not happy, you are not using your power in the right way. If you don't feel loved, you are not using your power in the right way. If you see your future as lacking hope, you are not using your power in the right way.

But, it is never too late to become what you hoped you might become.

FREE WILL

Have you ever seen the film, *The Truman Show*? Jim Carrey plays the central character, Truman Burbank, who lives his life without realising it is a set populated by actors. Truman didn't question anything until the true knowledge of his life was forced upon him.

At that point, he had to choose to stay in his secure existence knowing the truth or to exercise his free will and take a leap into the unknown. Happily, he chose the leap of faith.

We are all living our own version of Truman Burbank's life. We are all in our own kind of dream, or trance until one day you decide to wake up and look for new evidence that another world exists out there. Those who choose this path will find out that they are no longer a victim of circumstance but can make their own choices and thrive.

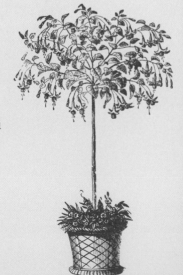

Whatever success or pain you have experienced in the past, it's in the past now.

'Freedom is what you do with what's been done to you.'

Jean-Paul Sartre

'When one realises one is asleep, at that moment one is already half-awake.'

P.D. Ouspensky

THE POWER OF THE UNIVERSE

All the power you will ever need to create a happy life is here right now. It is not outside but inside you.

There is always a route to happiness even in the most difficult of circumstances.

These two statements are universal truths but most of the billions of people on this planet are ignorant of them, even though every great sage throughout history has written about this for millennia.

Your true power is the power to manifest a different life. This power is contained here in the world we all live in and is available to you right now. We are and have always been powerful. This power is not something which we learn in a school or university. It is not something which a politician or priest can give us. This power is the gift of the universe to each of us when we are born.

Every sage in history has believed that there are two parts to the universe which are simultaneously in existence: the physical world and what is called the spiritual, energetic or metaphysical world. You have a physical body and an energetic body, which means you live simultaneously in both worlds even if you are only aware of your physical body the majority of the time.

The world is made up of atoms as indeed are you. Each and every atom in your body is the same as the atom in the universe. They are all made of a shared substance: light, also known as the creative life force. There are roughly 30 trillion cells in your physical body and each cell contains the life force of the universe inside it. You may *feel* separate from other things and people, but every thought you have and action you take creates change in the world around you because you are connected.

The life you have now is the one you co-created with the universe. As co-creator of this world with the life force of the universe, you can unmake it and remake it in accordance with what your heart truly wants to bring into being. Anything can be changed by intentionally directing your mind to what you want instead. By changing something in yourself, you will set off a reaction in everything around you and the world you live in will be fresh and new.

What you *do*, and what you *think* and *focus* on, influences every part of the universe: the spiritual and material. This means that you can deliberately influence your experience in the physical world.

The universe is ordered and logical. It obeys spiritual laws which are explained throughout the book. Through practising an ordered, intentional mental process which works with these laws and by learning the art of manifesting, you can create a new life for yourself. The universe will work with you to help you. When you set an intention to manifest anything: a new relationship, money, a home, etc. the power of your thought creates a change in the energetic world. The material world then immediately rearranges itself to bring what you desire into existence in accordance with the spiritual laws of the universe. Through the power of your intentional thought and focus, it will help you to change the material world you live in, and bring you new experiences, new feelings, new people and new things.

You have a partner in the universe who will never leave your side or let you down. There is nothing the universe cannot do for you. It has infinite unexpected ways of manifesting your desires into reality in the material world.

'The reason why the universe is eternal is that it does not live for itself; it gives life to others as it transforms.'

Lao Tzu

THE LAW OF ONENESS

We are all subject to spiritual laws. It doesn't matter
your age, or ethnicity or what country you live in.
These laws are universal and constant according to
the great masters. The first of these powerful laws is
the Law of Oneness. This law states that you are part
of the universe, not separate from it. Everything in
the universe is interconnected because it all springs
from the same source and is built from the same
life force. The material and spiritual realms are
joined as is everything in them: this includes things,
people, thoughts, and feelings. Although you live
in the material world, you can't see this connection,
nevertheless because we are all connected, everything
you do, think and feel impacts others around you.

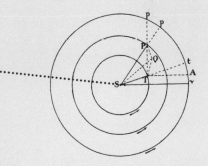

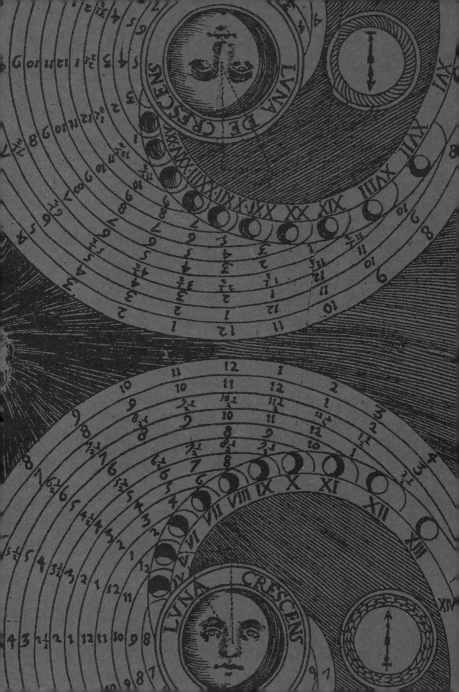

THE LAW OF ATTRACTION

The Law of Attraction is the next spiritual law of the universe. What it tells us is that *like attracts like*. In simple language, you attract into your life whatever you choose to focus on, consciously and unconsciously. Your thoughts and feelings put a vibration to the universe. From the moment you were born you have been the co-creator of your life whether you have been aware of it or not. Your partner in this process of creation is the force of the universe. Together with the universe, you create every moment of every day and everything that materialises in your life.

If you want to attract happiness you must attract it by vibrating on the same frequency as happiness. If you are loving you will attract love. But by being pessimistic or believing that life is tough, you will only attract more negative experiences. When you conceive of a new life, truly believe it will happen and start to act towards it, you begin to vibrate different thoughts to the universe and attract different experiences.

'There exists in nature … a force that would enable the man capable of seizing and directing it to change the face of the world. The will of intelligent beings acts directly on this light, and by means of it on all that part of Nature which is submitted to the modifications of intelligence. This light is the common mirror of all thoughts and all forms; it preserves the images of everything that has been, the reflections of past worlds, and, by analogy, the sketches of worlds to come.'

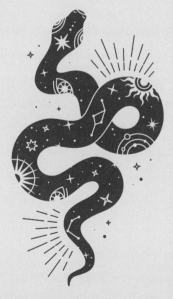

Éliphas Lévi

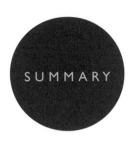

SUMMARY

You are subject to the Law of Oneness and are
connected to everything in the world.

❀

You are subject to the Law of Attraction and your
outer world reflects your inner world.

❀

Happiness is your right in this world.
You are born to be happy, not to suffer.

❀

Your past does not determine your future.

❀

All the power you will ever need to obtain
happiness is here now.

❀

It is only when you believe you are limited that you
will limit your personal power. You have FREE WILL
and can take control.

❀

Begin to CONCEIVE what you want and
BELIEVE you can have it.

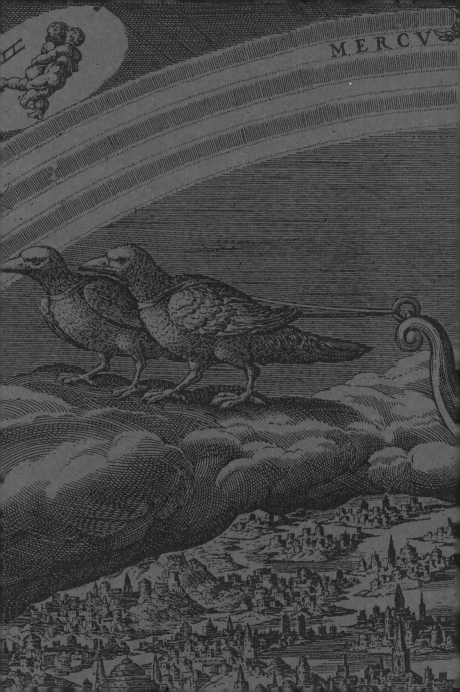

MERCV

CHAPTER TWO

DESIRE

'Imagination is the first step in creation, whether in words or trifles. The mental pattern must always precede the material form.'

William Walker Atkinson

One day a stonemason takes a chunk of marble and places it carefully in front of him. He looks at it and imagines what it can become. At first the only image that exists is in his imagination. Slowly he transfers the image from his mind's eye and imagines it coming into being. Each day he carves and carves deeper adding more detail until a perfect figure emerges from the stone.

This is the process of manifestation: to take what exists only in the imagination and impress it upon matter with thoughts and actions until it comes into reality.

You are the stonemason. Your tool is your imagination, and your material is the life force of the universe. What do you want to create?

'If we do not
know what port
we are steering
for, no wind is
favourable.'

Seneca

KNOW WHAT YOU WANT

The first step in the art of manifesting is to desire something. Think about these questions:

※ What do you want in your life?

※ Do you want to have something? Be something? Know something? Experience something? Do something? Let go of something you have already?

※ What is absent from your life which would make you happy?

※ What is present in your life which no longer makes you happy?

It's OK if you don't have answers to these questions

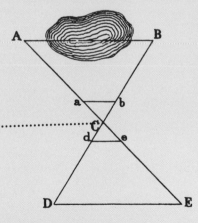

straight away. There is an awareness exercise in this chapter which will help you get in touch with what's important to you.

You are *always* manifesting whether you realise it or not. The difference when you learn how to manifest is to set about manifesting intentionally. The one thing you *can't* do is stop changing. This is not a static universe. Change always happens because we are all subject to the cycles and waves of the universe. It's important to say, of course many people find change uncomfortable but consider this: without change you could not live in this universe. The universe is made of energy and without energy you would not exist right now.

When you intentionally work out what will bring you happiness and state your desires to the universe you are no longer subject to what you are unconsciously manifesting. Instead, you can *have* what you want to *have* and *be* what you want to *be* and *do* what you want to *do*.

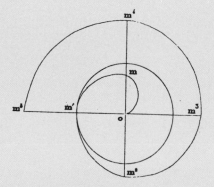

'Every man is maker of his own fortune.'

Albanian proverb

'If you do not change direction, you may end up where you are heading.'

Lao Tse

CHANGE YOUR EXPECTATIONS

Most people spend a lot of their power focusing on what they don't want.

The two lessons I was taught all those years ago about manifesting were:

What you focus on is what you will get.

What you resist will persist.

What this means is, you will create the world you expect to create.

Life is very precious. This is a wonderful world to live in if you know how you were always supposed to live in it. The world is full of beauty which is here for us to notice and experience. It is a gift, a privilege, and a miracle to live in the material world and experience life here. But, we don't always think of life in this way.

It is said that one of the most common regrets of the dying is that they wish they had had the courage to live a life true to themselves, not the life others expected of them. Another is that they wish they had allowed themselves to be happier.

It is easy to get distracted and side-tracked by life so much you forget to notice how extraordinary it is. Every time you complain about how terrible your life is: whether to a friend or to the dog, you are focusing on what you don't want. But if you keep *not* wanting things you will just create more of them. Focus instead on creating the life you have always wanted to live.

At some point this also means taking a leap of faith. Instinctively, most of us want evidence of what is to come before we believe it is coming. Many people won't take the risk of facing their lives in a new direction because they refuse to believe good is coming to them. It is only when the moment to change has passed and they look backwards that they see what might have been.

The leap of faith is to face life forwards with hope like that sculptor who sees what he wants to create and lets it grow in his imagination. When you are willing to do this, you are ready to manifest.

'If then, I were asked for the most important advice I could give, that which I considered to be the most useful to the men of our century, I should simply say: in the name of God, stop a moment, cease your work, look around you.'

Leo Tolstoy

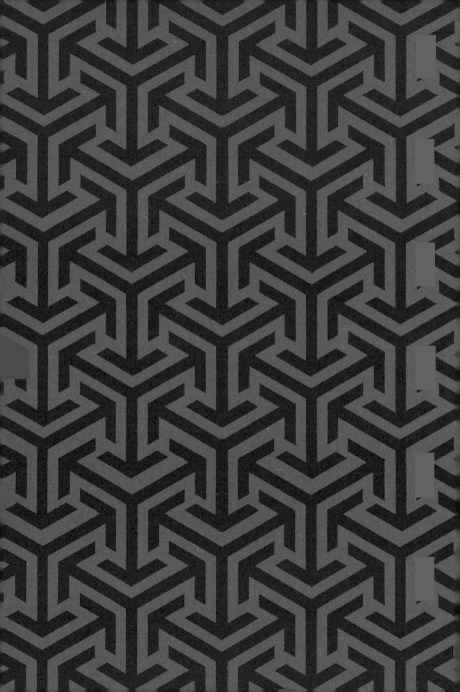

WHAT REALLY MATTERS TO YOU?

Human beings are always so busy. We rush around and don't take the space to really consider what's important. That's why so many of us accumulate possessions we don't really need or stay in jobs or relationships which don't satisfy or fulfil us. You could call this, living in the audience seats of life.

Living in the audience seats of life feels safe. It is easy to let life flow past and watch TV, or buy something new or hope for the workday to be over. It is particularly easy in modern life to spend a day researching the latest gadget or complaining about your relationship or gossiping with friends. The list of things we can choose to do is endless. Being busy can be addictive but it keeps us trapped in a small world.

When you rush around never allowing time to be still, you are focusing very narrowly. It's as if you're seeing life on a small phone screen. But around that screen there is more going on. When you are still and let your awareness open up, you give yourself the space to connect with your deepest desires. You notice the periphery: the corners and margins beyond the screen.

BUILDING AWARENESS

Here is a practice you can do for a few minutes to expand your awareness into the periphery and discover what's important to manifest.

Be still. Stop doing what you are doing and just simply close your eyes and breathe.

When you are still, your body relaxes, and your breath deepens.

Let your awareness open. If you don't focus on anything in particular, you will notice how your awareness shifts and expands by itself.

Now allow your awareness to expand to take in what is happening in the periphery. Become aware of your surroundings. Notice the sounds and smells and subtle changes in light even with your eyes closed. It's as if you are leaving the narrow focus of the small screen you were focusing on and seeing that there is infinite space around you.

Return your attention to your body. Imagine opening your head up and letting in the universal light so it floods your body with light. Allow this light to flow into the room or place you are in.

Expand your awareness and notice the light filling up the country you live in, then beyond this the whole world opens out in front of you filling with light.

Beyond this, the sun, moon, stars and the whole expanse of the universe fill with light.

Notice all the possibilities which exist in the world.

You haven't paid attention before because you were too busy paying attention to other things.

What do you really desire more than anything?

Allow any thoughts to come gently to you.

Now bring all that light from every corner of the universe back into your body and into your heart.

Open your eyes.

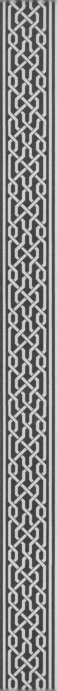

By taking the time to stop every day just for a few minutes and pay attention to the space around you, you are training yourself to notice more possibilities in your life. A few minutes a day may not seem much but can produce miracles.

As you practise awareness you will soon notice that your life has been a series of often unconscious choices. Isn't it time to look at this great big universe and make new choices? There are infinite paths you can take and each one can bring a new life full of joy and fulfilment. Now write down your first thoughts about what you desire to manifest.

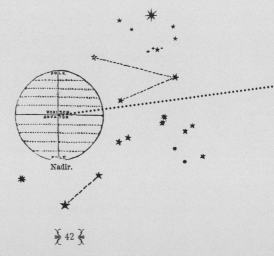

'Live life as
if everything
is rigged in
your favour.'

Rumi

AREAS OF YOUR LIFE

This second exercise is to get you thinking in a more conscious way about what you want to change.

Think about each area of your life. There are some categories written down below but you can add as many as you like.

Health
Relationships
Career
Life purpose
Wealth
Family
Spirituality

On a scale of one to ten, mark your levels of happiness in each area?

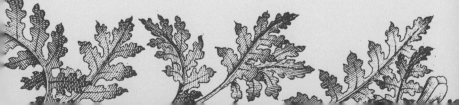

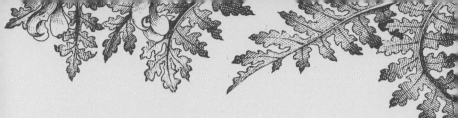

How balanced is your life?

Choose a significant birthday in the future. If your life carries on in the same way as you get older, what is likely to happen with your levels of happiness for each area at that age? In ten years? In twenty years?

When you picture this future, are you happy with what you see?

Which is the most important area for you and why?

What do you desire to change in each area of your life?

To do something? To be something? To have something? Write down what you want to bring into your life.

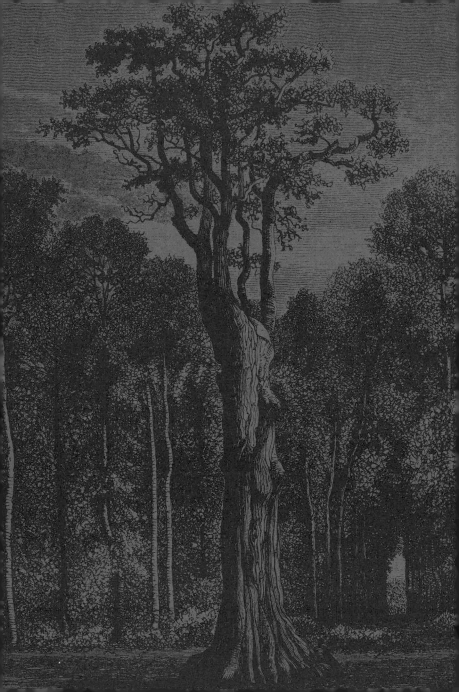

FORMULATING YOUR DESIRES

One you've started to work out what's important to you to change in your life, decide what you want to manifest. Write it down in a single sentence:

I desire xxxxxxxxxx

Now, again, STOP and double check.

Why do I want this?

What this often now reveals is a feeling, for example because you want love or happiness or fulfilment.

Then,

Is this desire the best means of getting this feeling? Or, is there something else even better I could manifest which could get me more of this feeling?

As soon as you are pretty confident what you want, it's important that you do one final check:

Is manifesting this in my life really important enough that I will make this the focus of my energy? Am I certain that this desire I have is good for me and those around me?

NEXT, TURN YOUR DESIRES TO AIMS

Now take what you have written and state it not as a desire but as an aim. When you write an aim you write it down as if it is *happening to you right now*.

For example,

I now have xxx

I am now xxx

I am now doing xxx

By writing your desire in the present tense using the word 'NOW', the universe recognises your desire as something to be brought into existence as soon as possible, rather than a *want* which can remain in the future. A want is just a hope, but an aim is a command to the universe to make it come true. A want is something we would like to have but don't necessarily expect to have. An aim written in the present tense tells your brain (and the universe) that you expect and intend to receive what you have written.

USE POSITIVE LANGUAGE

Do choose your words very carefully when you write down your aims. Think about the next two sentences:

I am not sad.

I am happy.

What picture do you have in your mind when you say each one? Only one of those sentences produces good feelings. When you say 'I am not sad', your brain still pictures sadness rather than happiness because of the negative phrasing.

Here's another example,

I won't have chocolate cake every day. I must not think of chocolate cake.

What are you picturing? Of course, chocolate cake.

If you wanted to give up chocolate cake you would need to think about what you would eat instead and formulate a sentence like,

I am eating lots of healthy fruit and vegetables every day.

Think about what you desire to manifest. If you have written something you *don't* want, change it to what you *do* want instead and make that want into an aim, for example:

I don't want to be homeless = I now have a home of my own.

I don't want a bad relationship = I now have a loving boyfriend.

I don't want this career anymore = I now have a job I love going to every day.

Of course, what you intend to manifest is still subject to laws of time and space. If you want to manifest a new car it is unlikely to fall from the sky in front of you. Not impossible but unlikely! Because of this, think about giving yourself some early evidence of success. Some people, when they start to write down what they want to manifest, document huge aims which are too distant and too big for them to succesfully manifest. It is fine to intend to create big changes, but when you first begin manifesting it is a good idea to create some smaller changes, so you see them happening more quickly. This will build your confidence as life changes step by step every day. Even small changes happening on a regular basis will alter the course of your life forever.

Revisit your manifesting aims. Once you are satisfied with what you have written get ready to allow the universe to work its magic as you learn the next steps to take in the art of successful manifesting.

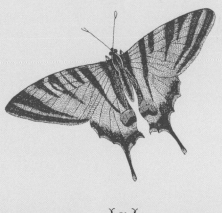

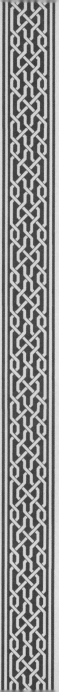

'Imagination is
the creative faculty
of the human
mind, the plastic
energy – the
Formative
Power.'

Dr William Westcott

THE LAW OF VIBRATION

The next spiritual law is the Law of Vibration. Can you remember a time when you thought, I'm really not on the same wavelength as this person?

What we mean by wavelength is the vibration a person gives out.

This is a vibrational universe. Everything in the universe is made up of energy vibrating at different speeds: atoms, molecules and quarks. Human beings also vibrate because we too are made up of the same substance.

You are like a magnet, attracting to you what you *are*. The things and events which come to you, positive and negative, are attracted by the emotional frequency and vibration of the thoughts and feelings you have. The universe responds *precisely* to this vibration and attracts a life full of experiences which exactly accord, with a one hundred percent match, to the vibration you put out.

This explains why people attract different

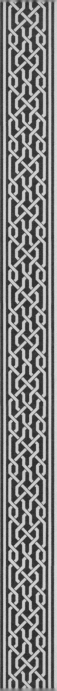

experiences in life. The person with a higher (positive) vibration will attract more positive experiences than someone with a lower (negative) vibration. You will also attract people with similar vibrations to you as your friends.

In other words, if you have a loving vibration, you will attract more love into your life. If your vibration lacks abundance you will experience scarcity and poverty in your life. If you think you are lucky, you will attract more luck.

The Law of Vibration also says you can raise or lower your vibration by changing your beliefs and thoughts and feelings, as well as the daily actions you take. If you want to manifest positive things in your life, then take positive actions that are good for you and others. Build into your life experiences anything that encourages positive emotions such as joy, gratitude, love, and compassion. Raise your vibration to exactly match the positive vibration of what you want to attract, and it will surely come.

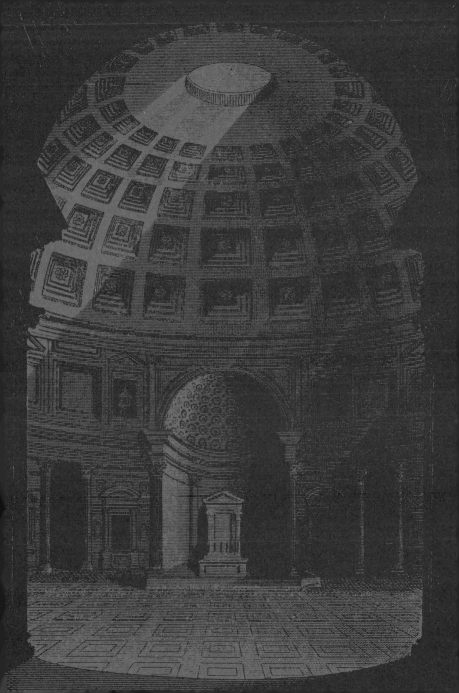

'The whole world is a very narrow bridge, and the main thing is to be totally unafraid.'

Rabbi Nachman of Breslov

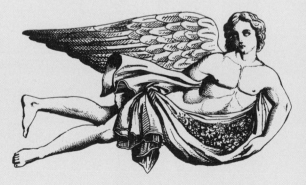

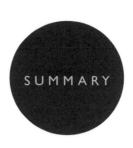

SUMMARY

Begin to dream of what you are
going to manifest.

❀

You are always changing, so focus on what
you want to change. There are infinite paths
you can choose at any point in your life.

❀

Think positive thoughts about what
you want, not negative thoughts about
what you don't want.

❀

Now turn your wants into AIMS.

❀

ASK for what you desire and state it in the
PRESENT TENSE as a command to the
universe to bring it into being. Imagine it is
here right NOW.

❀

The LAW OF VIBRATION will
attract change into your life when you
change your vibration.

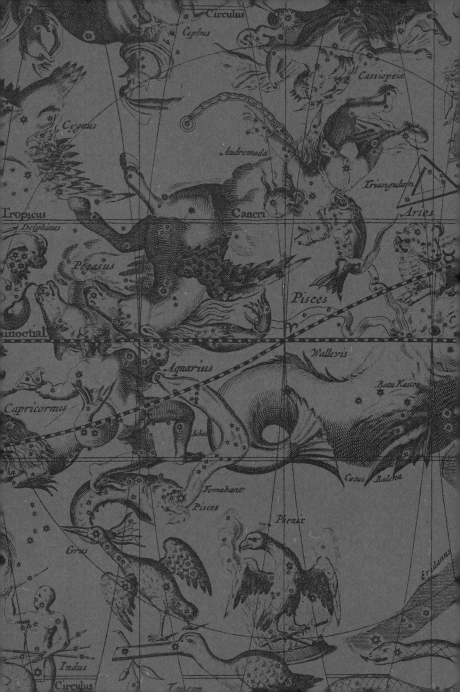

CHAPTER THREE

USE YOUR IMAGINATION

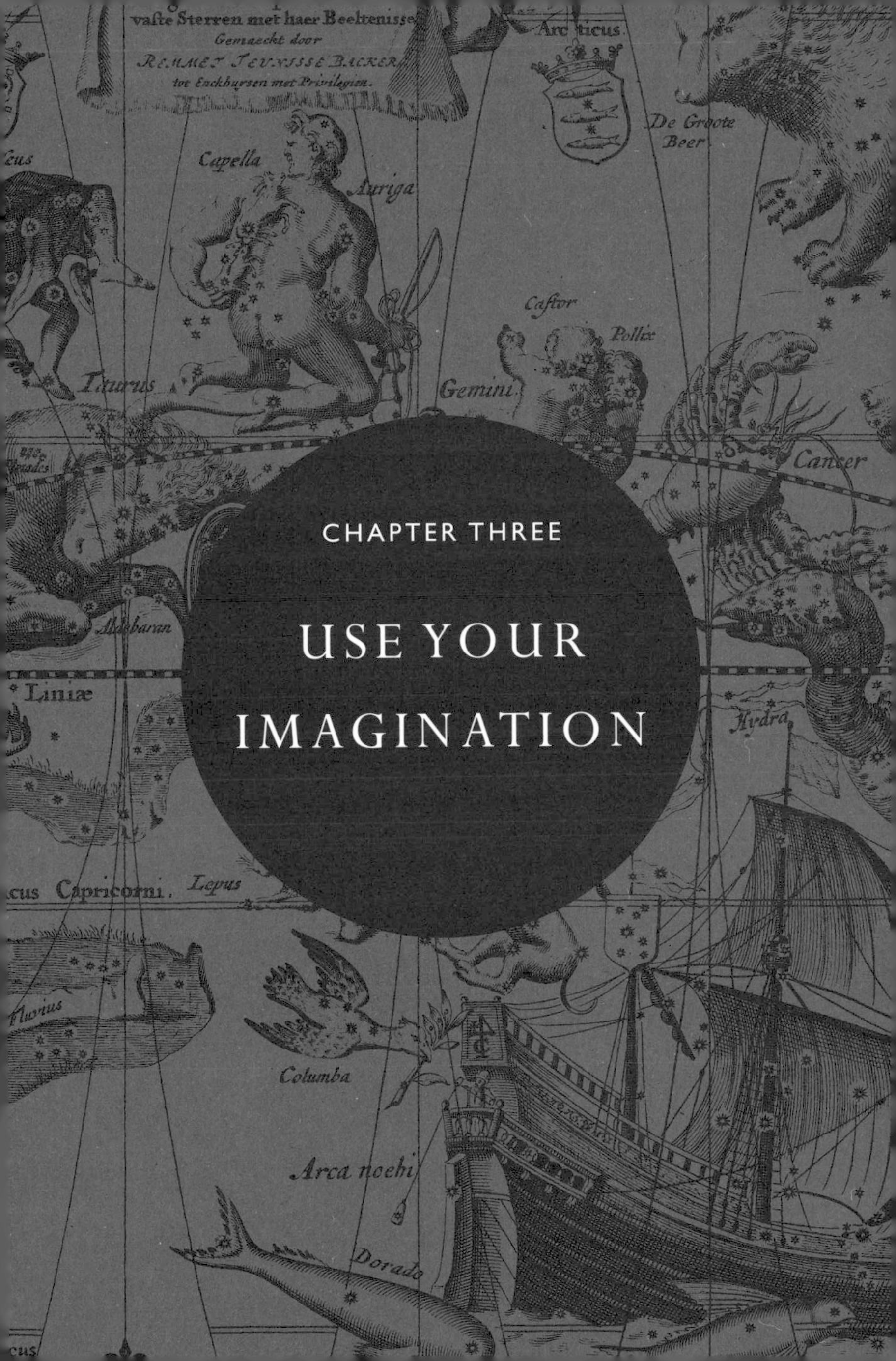

'The soul attracts that which it secretly harbours; that which it loves, and also that which it fears.'

James Allen

If this is your first time manifesting, like any new skill, it takes practice. If you haven't ever consciously practised manifesting before, you will need to hone your imagination to make your manifesting aims powerful. This will raise the vibration of your manifests and attract it in more quickly and accurately.

Think about one of the aims you wrote down. Do you have a clear picture of it in your mind's eye? Can you imagine it fully as if it exists in your universe right now? Is it a picture which makes you feel happy when you think about it?

If you can picture what you aim to create and can see it and feel what it will be like when you manifest it then you are ready to manifest successfully.

If on the other hand, you don't have a clear picture or a good feeling when you think about your aim, then you need to get your imagination fired up.

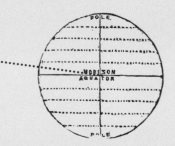

THE POWER OF YOUR TWO
MINDS COMBINED

You have two minds: your conscious mind (your left brain / willpower) and your subconscious mind (your right brain / imagination). Manifesting only works if both minds are fully aligned. Together your two minds look after your spiritual, mental, physical and emotional wellbeing. But the greater actor is your subconscious. You cannot manifest a change successfully with willpower alone.

When you state your intention to manifest something to the universe, the universe should obey you. However, it's only going to obey your instructions if both minds are in agreement, otherwise no matter what you wrote down, it won't believe you really intend to create it. To change your life, you need to know how to give precise instructions to your subconscious in the language of your imagination so you can manifest what you want now.

This is how it works. Your conscious mind (your will) is like the captain of a ship. It determines what you want and

what you intend.
It sends out a
command to the
crew. Think of your
subconscious mind
(your imagination) as your
ship's crew. Your crew takes
the instructions the captain has
given them and starts to steer the ship in
the right direction but only if the instructions are
clear. If your picture of what you intend to manifest is
wishy washy or has negative feelings attached, your crew
is going to revert to its previous instructions and refuse
to steer the ship forward.

How can you align your two minds? Firstly, by
ramping up the positive feelings around your aims.
Your subconscious will respond to pleasurable feelings,
so if you make a picture of what you want and imagine
having it with lots of good feelings attached then your
subconscious will do its best to help manifest it. When
you state your desire, your subconscious immediately
asks, 'Will that really make me happy?'

If the answer is 'no' then it will stop it happening.

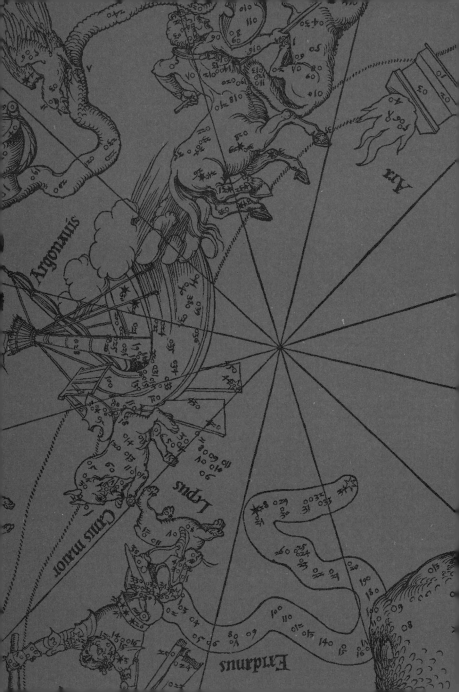

This is because your subconscious acts as your inner protector. It will always steer your ship to what it sees as the safest destination which is generally the one you are most familiar with.

Your subconscious will always choose what it thinks will *feel* best for you, even if you don't *consciously* think it's the better choice.

Secondly, you need to get really good at making pictures of what you want. You can practise this by creating vision boards, cutting out pictures of the sort of future you want or just practising using your imagination.

You will learn how to impress your desires and intentions on your subconscious mind so that it can work for you below the surface to manifest your desires.

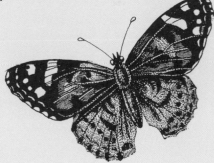

THE ROLES OF THE SUBCONSCIOUS

Your subconscious runs and heals the body, stores memories and produces feelings.

It is the home of our intuition and instincts. It runs according to the directions we give it.

Your subconscious is telepathic.

Your subconscious is your imagination.

It doesn't think in words but in pictures, symbols and feelings.

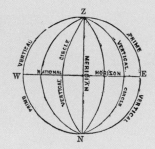

'One picture is worth a thousand words.'

Chinese proverb

IMAGINING A BALLOON

Here is a demonstration of how powerful your imagination is.

- ❈ Hold your two hands out parallel in front of you with your palms facing upwards. Close your eyes.

- ❈ Imagine I am placing a pile of heavy books on your right hand. Feel how heavy your hand is with the weight of the books on top of it.

- ❈ Now look at your left hand in your mind's eye. See that I am tying a balloon to your left wrist. You can feel it floating up in the air with the lightness of the balloon pulling your hand up as the balloon floats higher and higher.

- ❈ Now open your eyes and see how your hands have separated. The right hand is lower than the left.

You did this through the power of your imagination.

IMAGINING A LEMON

Here is a second demonstration of how when you imagine something vividly, your subconscious treats it as if it is real.

- ❀ Close your eyes.

- ❀ Imagine a lemon in front of you.

- ❀ Now take an imaginary knife and slice the lemon into quarters. Take a quarter of the lemon and put it into your mouth.

- ❀ Suck the lemon and notice how your mouth becomes dry.

The reason the lemon and balloon demonstrations work is because your imaginary lemon and balloon feel and look real in your mind and the unconscious accepts that neither are going to harm you. When you picture your aim, you must see and feel it in as much detail as in these last two exercises.

'Be careful what
you wish for, you
will receive it.'

Anonymous

CREATE A FUTURE MEMORY

Now you've demonstrated to yourself how effective your imagination is, you can learn how to transfer your aim into your subconscious by creating a rich picture. We call this a *future memory* or *future piece of evidence*. It should be clear enough that when you eventually manifest what you want you will think, I remember putting that into my imagination and now I've got it!

✺ Take the piece of paper on which you have written down your aim.

✺ Sit down and relax (see the next chapter for tips).

✺ Think of a clear image of what you want.

✺ When you reach the time when this really does manifest in your life, will you know it has happened? (That sounds like a stupid question but if you're not clear enough you may not recognise your successes).

✺ Be precise and think of what the picture which will let you know you have manifested your desire will be. This picture should be clear and specific so will recognise the moment when you get it. (For example, perhaps it is you on your wedding day, the moment you kiss your partner as the celebrant has just told you that you are married. Maybe it is the moment you receive a key to your new home, or taking a call and hearing your future employer say you have the new job. Perhaps, it is you standing in front of a mirror seeing your washboard abs!)

* Build the picture in your mind. It may be a still or moving picture, framed or unframed, large or small, vivid or dull. Generally, it helps to turn up the colours and make the picture larger, so it impresses on your imagination.

* Think of what colours are in the image, what are the sounds in your picture, the tastes and smells? Is there music or anyone speaking in your picture?

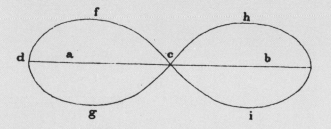

'You are today where your thoughts have brought you; you will be tomorrow where your thoughts take you.'

James Allen

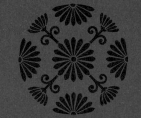
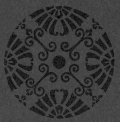

The first time I wanted to write a book, I imagined the exact words the publisher would say to me, and they rang me up a year later and used those very same words. The second manifest which was successful for me involved me buying my home. I visualised holding the key in my hand as the estate agent handed it to me and placing it in the door as my partner said to me, 'We've finally got the home we always wanted.' I also imagined exactly what the home would look like inside and I got what I had imagined, down to the words my partner said to me.

RAMPING UP THE FEELING

The next part of picturing your desire and turning it into a manifestation is to create lots and lots of positive *feeling* around it.

This part is so important. You can only get your aim with positive consequences if you have great future feelings associated with it. Your imagination is not just visual: it responds to all the senses.

As you see the picture of you with your desired outcome, deliberately fill your body with positive emotions such as joy and excitement, as if you have got exactly what you wanted.

MANIFESTING STORIES

RHIANNA

Rhianna really wanted to be slim, and set a desire in July to reach her target weight by September of the same year. It didn't work. When we discussed what had happened, it was clear that although she had written out her desire and visualised what she wanted, she was yearning for her favourite chocolate cake every day and associated dieting with pain. This was a simple job for her subconscious: pleasure from chocolate cake now versus pleasure from future weight loss plus pain of dieting. The only way Rhianna could overcome this was to ramp the positive feelings when she visualised her desire.

TED

Ted aimed to be successful in business but was scared working hard would be bad for his health. Of course, his subconscious kicked in to protect his health. Every time he got near his goal of building his company he got the feeling he was making too big a sacrifice and failed to meet his financial targets again and again because he wasn't willing to go the extra distance – in his case staying extra hours at the office. He only overcame this when he visualised a different career which balanced health and success by taking on a business partner to share the workload.

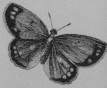

ESME

Esme was an attractive thirty-nine-year-old manager who had worked for years in the retail industry. When I met her she had been in a long term relationship with Paulo who didn't want to marry her. She had good friends but couldn't bring herself to leave Paulo even though she was increasingly unhappy because of her fear of 'ending up alone'. When we discussed what made her feel like this she said, 'No one I know has met a partner at this age.' We spent some time discussing what she wanted instead of what she didn't want and she wrote a list of desires and visualised them.

A few months later, she had the courage to leave Paulo, she spent some time by herself and started internet dating. Gradually, she became open to the new evidence that there were many good men out there. A year later, Esme was happily engaged to Rafael, a forty-year-old man she met at work. It turned out there had been someone nearby all along. Once her eyes were open she found him.

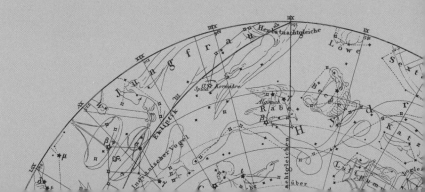

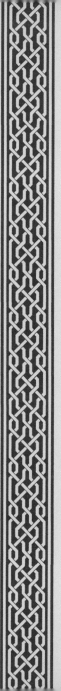

THE LAW OF CORRESPONDENCE

The Hermetic saying is: 'As above so below. As within, so without.' The spiritual Law of Correspondence says that our outer world is an exact reflection of our inner world. The personal world you live in is the world you have helped to create and all the power you will ever need to change it is in your possession right now. It is not contained in some secret box in a different part of the universe nor in the past or in a future you. If your outer world is full of chaos, it is because your inner world is full of chaos. To change your future simply change your focus and the universe will change around you.

Each of us from birth builds a unique idea of reality: a subjective universe based on our millions of different experiences. Sometimes the picture you have of the world is not a helpful one so the universe you create is not the one you want to create. When we are

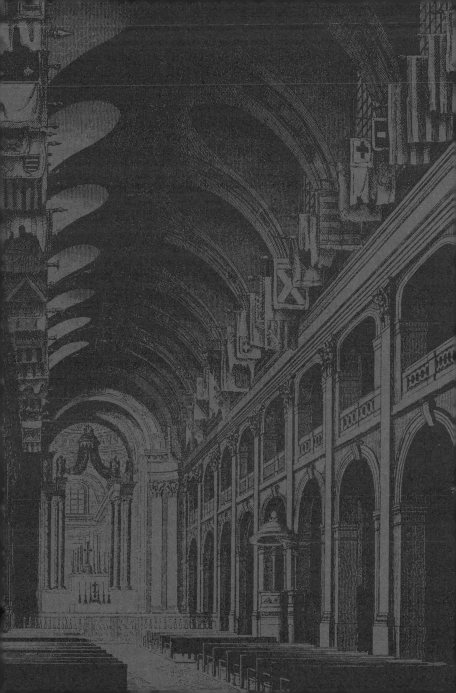

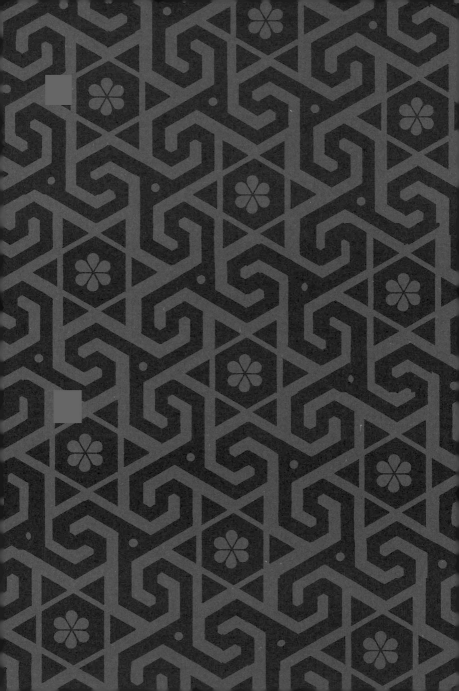

children, we often accept without question what we hear adults tell us or take other people's experiences as things which will inevitably come true for us as well. But these are not facts. The things you were told by adults as a child may not be helpful to you now. Without a change of consciousness, they stick in your subconscious mind and mean that you don't manifest what you want to manifest as an adult.

Choose the focus of your thoughts and change your future.

Think positive thoughts and you will manifest positive experiences. Take positive actions and you will manifest positive things. Speak positively about people and you will manifest positive relationships.

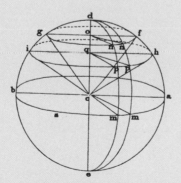

THE LAW OF REVERSED EFFECT

The Law of Reversed Effect tells us the harder you try to do something, the worse the result you get. Why? Because trying implies assumption of failure. If you feel you have to work hard to get a result you don't really believe in manifesting. You may think you believe in manifesting but if you are struggling it is a sign that your two minds are not aligned. Manifesting is an effortless process which happens when your conscious and subconscious work in harmony with each other.

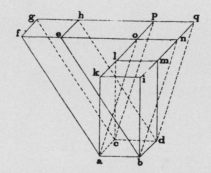

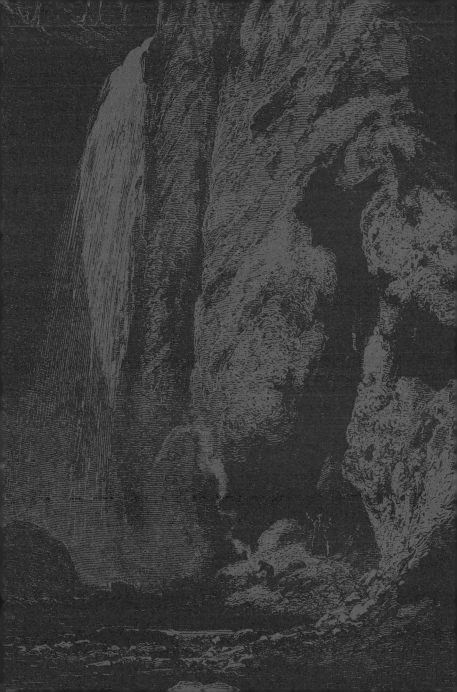

MANIFESTING STORY

BELLE

'One year, I imagined a trip to Malaysia taking place in the summer of the following year. I had been there before so I had a clear picture in my mind of sitting in a café I knew. I didn't mention it to anyone because I wasn't attached to the idea. I even forgot about it until one day a business colleague asked if I could come to do some translation work in Malaysia in June. We drank martinis at the café just as I had imagined.'

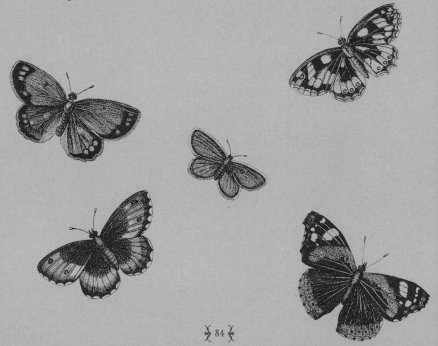

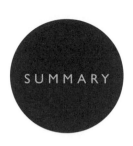

SUMMARY

You have two minds: your conscious mind (WILL) and your subconscious mind (IMAGINATION). To master manifesting you must align both minds with your desire.

✳

Consciously state what you desire. IMAGINE the exact moment you manifest your desire.

✳

Your subconscious will take that instruction and do its best to deliver it but only if you have communicated in a way it understands: through pictures, senses and feelings.

✳

Practise using your imagination to make pictures. Build a picture for your future memory of what your new reality looks like. Build as many details in as you can. Add colour and movement. Add sounds and tastes and smells.

✳

FEEL how good it will be when it happens.

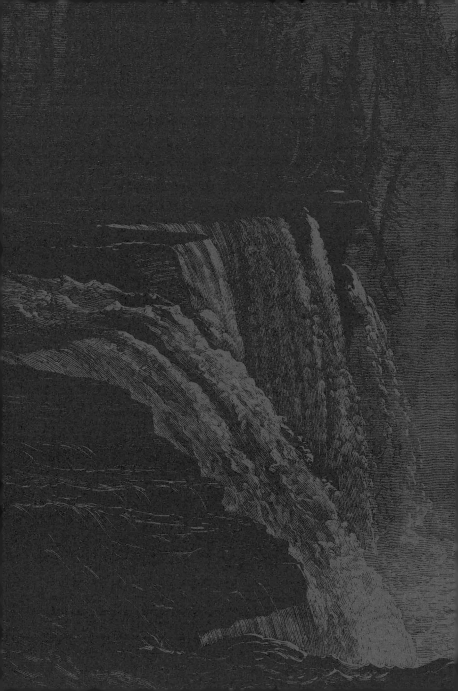

CHAPTER FOUR

RELAX

'To a mind that is still, the entire universe surrenders.'

Zhuangzi

RELAX

When you slow down and relax, you change. The world around you seems to become slower as your breath deepens and slows. Your brainwaves slow, and in scientific terms, you access what is called the alpha state. This is a powerful manifesting state.

ALPHA STATE

In normal life when you are going about your daily business your brainwaves are typically showing activity between fourteen and thirty Hz. In alpha state, your brain wave activity slows down to between seven and fourteen Hz. This is a state you will fall in and out of during the day even when you are not trying to relax. We access alpha state when we are daydreaming and also when falling asleep. Any kind of relaxation, meditation, hypnosis or self-hypnosis can take you into alpha state.

Hypnotists help their patients to access alpha state because in this state you are less critical, more open and more imaginative. In other words, there is more right-brain activity going on because you have good communication with your subconscious mind.

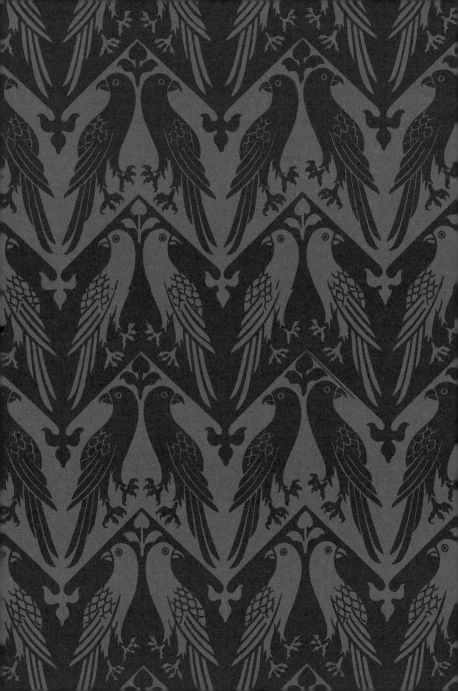

STILLNESS

By deliberately practising stillness, you train yourself
to access the alpha state when you want to. There are
many benefits to this when you are learning to manifest:
becoming aware of higher frequencies, expanding your
consciousness and creativity, as well as accessing your
intuition and inner truth. Most importantly, manifesting
your desires works best when you visualise them in a
relaxed state and *feel the positive feelings* you will have
when you attain your desire.

Stillness stops you rushing around and being busy.
It gives you a gap in your day when you can get in touch
with the moment and live absolutely in the here and
now. Being busy is a way of avoiding being in touch with
your feelings but as a master manifester you want to be
in touch with your feelings.

Stillness allows the deepest communication with
the subconscious which is why hypnosis starts with
an instruction to relax. In these moments of deep
relaxation, you can find the space to identify what you
feel and think, and to overcome false and negative
feelings and inner obstacles.

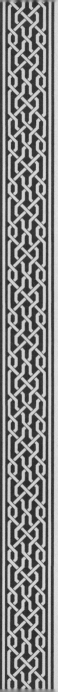

By finding space within yourself, your awareness is heightened. Some traditions believe that in order to communicate effectively with your higher self, you need to raise your frequency.

They believe that the physical world as a whole has a denser, heavier vibration, so if you want to you tap into the highest frequencies of the life force which exists in the lighter spiritual world, you must raise your vibration. Stillness does this and through stillness you will attract more precise manifesting.

Stillness also reminds us of the moment we are in.

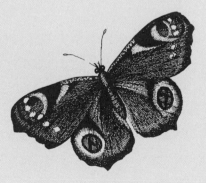

BREATHE

You are a breathing being and your breath is incredibly powerful. In the material universe, it is the breath which determines whether we live or die. Deepening and controlling the breath through practising relaxation can pull miracles towards you by changing the vibration you put out to the universe.

By taking a deep breath and noticing this moment right now, you can access beautiful feelings of inner peace.

Being in the now is also powerful as a tool for change. By changing your state and accessing alpha you have control of your emotions and the pictures you make in your mind.

You can access your feelings about the past and the future, and change the pictures you have of events in the past as well as future memories. This means just by relaxing and breathing deeply you can learn to let go of bad thoughts about the past or beliefs which hold you back, and you can change your future.

RELAX NOW

This is a simple relaxation method to begin with.

To relax, you simply sit and close your eyes. Notice your breathing. Notice where your breath is in your body. As you just let go, your breath will slow and deepen effortlessly. As your breath deepens, your body will relax.

* Let your breath naturally settle down. Your mind quiets down. There is no need to do anything, no need to be anywhere. You only need to allow your body to relax, as you rest your hands gently in your lap.

* Notice your head, face and neck relaxing.

* Notice your chest relaxing,

* Notice your arms and hands relaxing,

* Notice your stomach relaxing,

* Notice your legs relaxing.

- ※ As you relax, you sink into balance with the universe. As you relax more and more, you can allow good feelings to surface.

- ※ To go deeper count backwards from one hundred to one, telling yourself you are going deeper. As you reach one you will find yourself in a deep alpha state and in this state you can visualise clearly whatever you want.

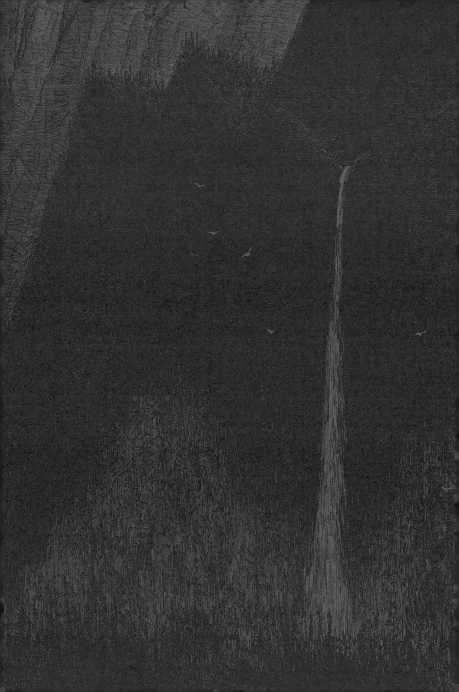

SECOND RELAXATION METHOD

※ Sit with your back and legs supported so you are comfortable, or if you prefer, you can lie down. Close your eyes.

※ Take a deep breath in… hold it… and breathe out.

※ Repeat this deep breath two more times.

※ When you breathe out, allow your body to release any tension it is holding so you can settle down and deeply relax.

※ Notice with interest how your body knows perfectly how much breath to take in and how much to take out in order for you to relax.

※ Now imagine in your mind's eye that you are holding a ball between your hands.

※ In your imagination, squeeze the ball as hard as you can until you can't squeeze it any harder. Then let go and allow yourself to drop down into deep relaxation.

POSTING YOUR AIM TO
THE UNIVERSE

Here is an extra step you can add to boost your manifesting power once you have mastered relaxing. This posting your aim method works as powerful symbolism for your subconcious.

⁕ First relax into the alpha state.

⁕ As you become still and centred, picture what you desire.

⁕ See the picture you imagined of the moment you have achieved your manifest as a present reality. As every detail becomes sharp and focused and you feel what you will be feeling as you finally manifest what you wrote down, imagine you are seeing the whole scene as if it is through your own eyes.

⁕ Now switch perspective.

⁕ In your mind's eye, step out of the scene you are visualising and see the same scene as if you are experiencing it like a viewer watching a film. See yourself in the picture feeling the happy emotions as you realise your manifest.

※ At this moment, freeze the picture and imagine holding it in your hands like a framed photograph.

※ Imagine floating up above your future and seeing below you the exact time you wish to manifest this.

※ Now drop the picture down into your future.

※ See in your mind's eye your whole future rearrange itself as it changes to take account of this new 'future memory' you will manifest.

※ Thank the universe in advance for bringing it to you.

※ Open your eyes.

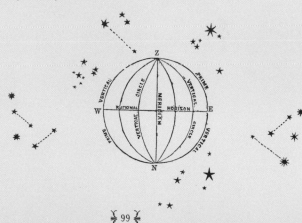

LETTING GO

By doing this exercise and dropping the picture into your future, you are telling the universe, I trust you to do what you need to do to make this happen even if I can't see the method.

It reminds you to let go of over-attachment to what you desire to manifest.

It may seem illogical but over-attaching to a desire will cause it NOT to manifest. The reason is that over-wanting something is actually doubting the universe's ability to deliver without involving your willpower.

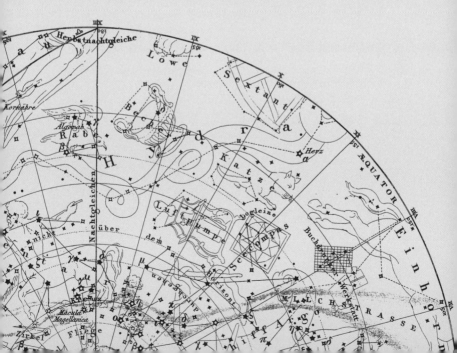

Letting go is the ONLY way it can happen. Letting go then taking action towards what you want tells the universe, I trust you and I will show my commitment.

Silence is very powerful. Avoid telling others what you intend to manifest. Over-talking about something can dilute that power because it is another way of over-attaching.

Instead, once you intend to manifest something, start building new habits to support it happening. Feel your excitement or delight at the accomplishment of your desire. Tear up any pieces of paper you wrote your aims on. Keep them alive in your imagination or as pictures on a vision board and commit to them through action.

'Life is a
balance of
holding
on and
letting go.'

Rumi

SPIRITUAL LAW 6
THE LAW OF TIME AND CREATION

In the spiritual universe there is no time. The past, present and future all exist simultaneously. The only time is the present moment.

The idea of time only exists in the mind. Past and future only exist as ideas. Think about something in the past? A memory will come to your mind. Think about something in the future? A picture of how you expect your future to be will come to your mind. Both the past memory and the future memories may be accompanied by feelings of happiness or anxiety, sadness, joy or other emotions. These feelings are kept alive by the pictures we store in our subconscious minds. The only time which really exists is right now, and therefore in the present we can create future memories as well as store past memories and the universe will treat them both as real.

MANIFESTING STORIES

JACK

'I set up a vision board and cut out lots of pictures from magazines of my future life. One of them was a picture of a black and white cat sitting in the sun. Two months later my neighbours moved and offered me their four-month-old black and white kitten who just happens to have exactly the same markings as the cat in the picture.'

TREV

'I woke up one morning with a strong sense I wanted to write again after not writing for more than a year. I opened my laptop and began writing. I laid out the chapters and wrote my opening introduction. Only three weeks later, my publisher approached me suggesting I write the very book I was working on.'

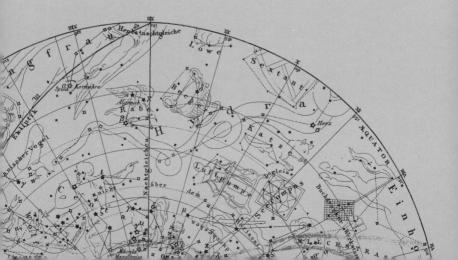

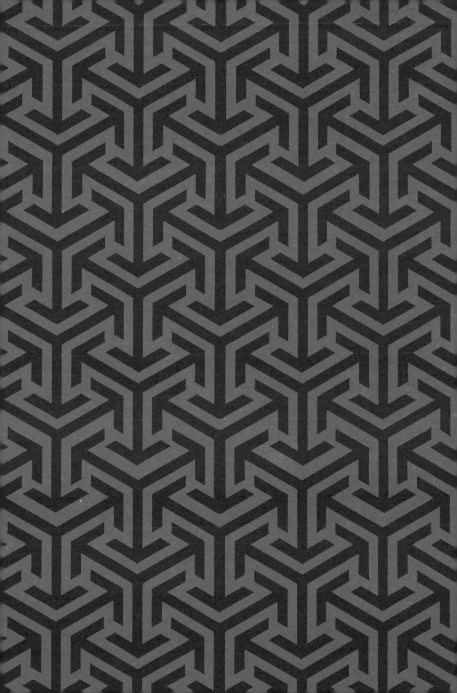

'Truth is not something outside to be discovered, it is something inside to be realised.'

Osho

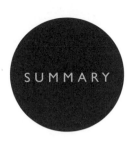

SUMMARY

RELAX: learn to practise regular
relaxation so you can access the
powerful ALPHA STATE.

✳

In this state visualise in detail
what you desire.

✳

Use the power of the alpha state
to POST your desire to the
universe.

✳

LET GO and trust.

✳

Keep silent about what you
intend to manifest.

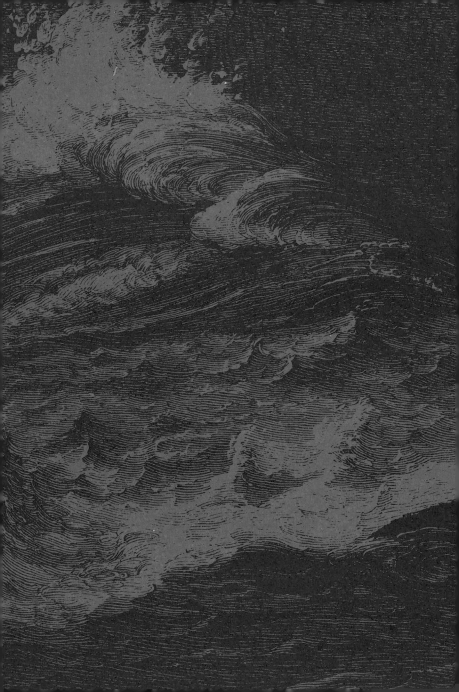

CHAPTER FIVE

COMMITMENT

'Do not wait. The time will never be "just right". Start where you stand, and work with whatever tools you may have at your command, and better tools will be found as you go along.'

Napoleon Hill

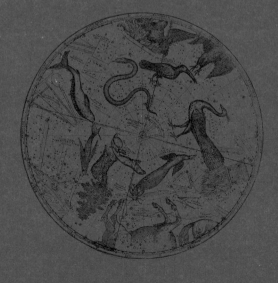

When a seed is planted in the ground in spring we don't see what goes on under the earth but we trust it will emerge as a plant in summer if we give it good soil and water to grow.

This is the same process by which manifesting works. First visualise, then trust, and finally act.

You have decided what you want to manifest, imagined it in colour and with feeling, and posted it to the universe. Now commit to your desire.

Commitment is the foundation of all achievement. Without commitment there are wants and hopes and aspirations but no change.

Commitment shows the universe you believe in what you are going to manifest. Commitment means taking actions daily which align with your stated aims.

If for example, you aim to manifest a new partner, don't turn down dates. If you aim to create a few friendships, accept invitations. What you manifest may come eventually in a different way, but you are showing the universe you are committing.

TAKE ACTION TODAY

Commitment means action. Show the universe you mean business every single day.

For example, if you want a new job, at some point you need to look at job adverts. If you want to climb Everest one day, have you started training?

For everything you wish to manifest, think of a first step you can take in the right direction however small. You don't need to know how you are going to get to the end point, just what you are going to do to start.

In fact, when you are trying to work out whether you really want this change in your life, ask yourself this revealing question: *will I do whatever it takes to manifest this?* (Let's assume whatever it takes is moral and ethical and good for you and the universe as a whole.)

Answering this question is incredibly helpful to get to grips with what's really important to you and for you to understand what part of your inner world you are not willing to change.

For example, if you need to work on your beliefs about love to manifest a loving partner, would you?

If you need to cold call to help you manifest the right job, would you?

With every action you take you will find your portfolio of successful manifests grows and this in turn, will provide evidence to your subconscious that you have mastered the art of manifesting. That will then feed through to even greater success in future manifesting.

Think about what you are going to manifest next. State to yourself: *I will apply all my power to making my desired aim come true.*

Think about even a tiny step which will point you in the right direction, and state to yourself: *As a first step, I will...*

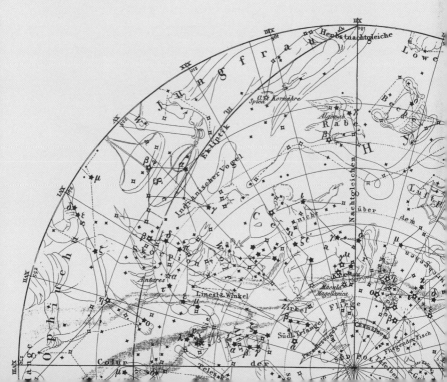

'Always bear in mind that your own resolution to success is more important than any other one thing.'

Abraham Lincoln

TAKING A LEAP OF FAITH

How much do you trust your ability to manifest what you've visualised?

In the 1700s the English writer Dr Samuel Johnson famously kicked a stone to prove that it was real and made of matter. This is the way most of us are taught. If it exists now it is real. If you can kick it then of course it exists.

But manifesting takes a leap of faith because it involves creating future memories you can't kick! You need to believe that the stone which doesn't yet exist in your material universe can soon exist. When you dream it, it's as if it exists in dream form waiting to drop into the material universe.

Trust is a vital part of commitment. Doubt will stop you manifesting because it turns your intentions back into wants and hopes again. The rule of a leap of faith is to believe *BEFORE* you have the material evidence in front of you. The pictures you form in your imagination have to be so real to you that you trust them.

Manifesting requires us to believe that the seeds of desire we plant will be worked on by a force outside our conscious awareness according to the spiritual laws of attraction, cause and effect, correlation, and vibration. You cannot force a manifest into existence with willpower and ego. Your will can only create a clear desire and blueprint for what you want and then set the manifest into motion. The force which does the manifesting is the life force of the universe, not your ego or will.

One of the ways to build trust in yourself is to manifest small results first rather than going for the biggest thing you desire. In this way you can create a trail of trust; paying attention to the evidence of your own successes.

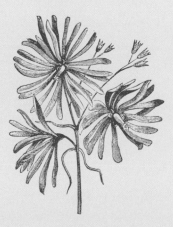

GRATITUDE

Thank you.

When you posted your aim to the universe, you said 'thank you in advance' for the universe delivering.

Be still for a moment and *feel* the words. Let the feeling resonate through your body. Saying thank you is one of the most powerful forces in the universe. Gratitude is the water for the seeds of desire you have planted in the life force of the universe.

When you say the words 'thank you' with real meaning and feeling, your gratitude will pull what you desire to manifest towards you because it tells the universe, 'I trust you.'

As with all the steps to manifesting, being grateful, saying thank you, and believing it as you say it takes practice if you aren't used to doing it.

The best way to learn real gratitude is to practise daily. It may not be that anything big has happened to you or come your way today.

That doesn't matter. Start small. Be grateful for the food you ate today. Be grateful for the people you have in your life even if they are far away. Be grateful for sleeping in a bed inside a warm room. Be grateful for your health even if it is imperfect.

Make a list of all the things you are grateful that you already have in your life. This lets the universe know you are grateful for every day you live. Be grateful for everything, even the bills you get.

Everything we experience gives us a gift even the difficult situations. If you can feel the gratitude this will shift your energy in an extraordinary way.

Now you can tell the universe what you are grateful for having, doing and being in the future. Make your list and feel the gratitude for what is about to manifest. This is how you can attract miraculous manifestation in your life.

GRATITUDE PRACTICE

Practise gratitude by focusing on what you are grateful for on a daily basis.

Each day, consider, 'What am I grateful for today?' Think of three things you are grateful for.

You can take this one stage further by thinking, 'How did I positively contribute to this uplifting experience / success happening?'

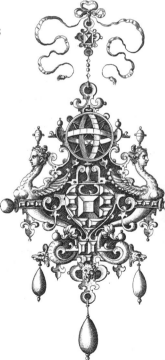

For example, 'I smiled at that person and they smiled back.' 'I learnt to cook and I am grateful for the food that tasted good today.' 'I exercised and now I am grateful for the good health I have as a result.'

When you get used to doing this you can add an additional practice.

Every night, thinking about what you manifested, say:

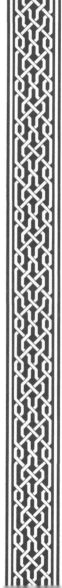

- ☼ *Thank you for this today.*

- ☼ *Thank you for that yesterday.*

- ☼ *Thank you for this tomorrow.*

When you say thank you for something which hasn't happened, you tell the universe you expect it to happen. By feeling good feelings about what you are experiencing, what you have already experienced and what you expect to experience, you will manifest good things every day.

Become grateful for bigger and better things every day and your manifests can become more and more powerful.

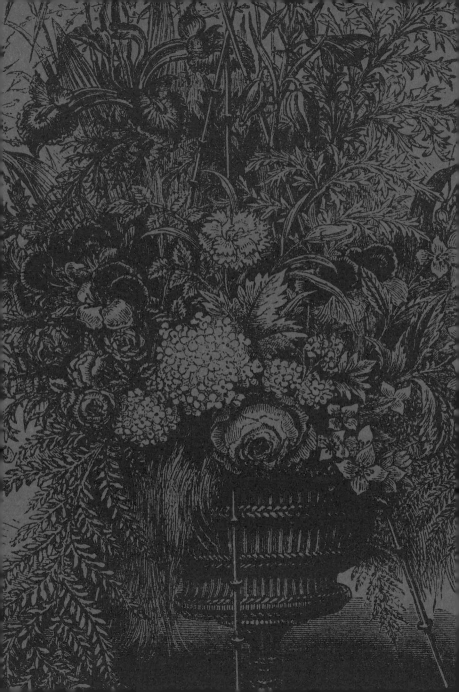

THE LAW OF ABUNDANCE

The Law of Abundance says that if we think and act with abundance we will be rewarded with more from the infinite source.

The best way to invite abundance is to be grateful for what you have already. If you focus only on what you don't have, you will produce thoughts of lack and the vibration of this thought form will produce more lack.

ABUNDANCE THINKING

There are some people in the world who are truly abundant. They may be the stranger who gives you directions in a strange city when you are lost, the friend who lends you an ear when you are sad, or the mother who hugs you when you need comfort. They may be the acquaintance who buys you a present and remembers your birthday or the relative who drives you to the hospital or who helps you out with a loan when you are in financial trouble. Abundance takes many forms.

They don't look for praise or good feedback. They don't keep a running total of the kindnesses they do for others in the expectation of payment in kind or in another form. These people are truly abundant. By being abundant with friends, family and strangers, they receive back from the universe in many different forms. It could be in the form of a favour, material reward or love; the greatest gift the universe can give.

Giving and receiving appear to be opposite but they are two ends of the same whole. The fastest way to receive what you want from the universe is to live abundantly.

Abundance thinking is essential to manifesting. If you manifest with a win-lose mentality you will stay in feelings of lack and poverty thinking. Your manifests will only give you partially good results. Instead, act as if the universe will bring you what you need.

Avoid conditional giving. Conditional giving is widespread. We run unconscious balance sheets: I gave this to her so I should get this back. I put this much effort into my manifest so it should be due to me now. If you attach strings or over-expectation to what you desire to manifest, it repels the result. Give your love and kindness freely without placing conditions on how much you give. Give freely without expectation and the universe will give freely to you.

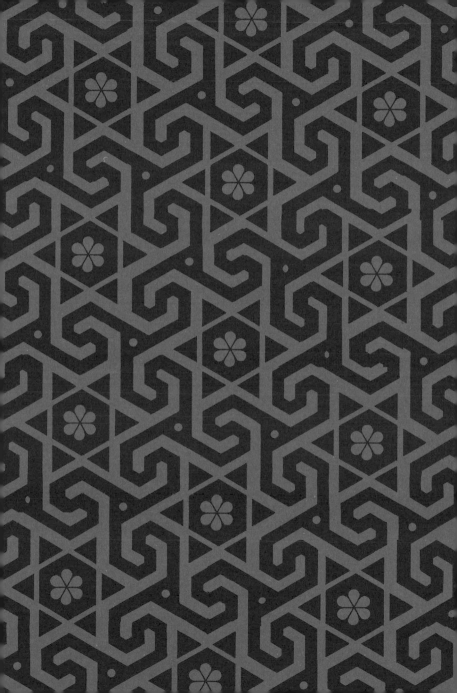

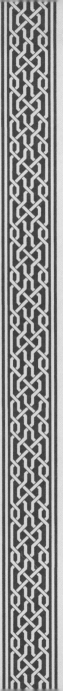

ACCEPT

You know how to say thank you. Now be ready to accept when the manifest appears.

Each day we receive countless gifts from the universe: the sun shining down, the breath in our bodies, friendship, perhaps a new opportunity in our life. Yet despite this experience of daily gifts, for some, giving is not the block but the ability and expectation of receiving are the biggest obstacles to manifesting effectively.

The universe is ALWAYS prepared to give to us if we are ready to receive it. Often you only notice years later that you didn't recognise the opportunities the universe was offering you or you didn't appreciate the material gifts you were offered.

When you find it hard to receive, it can be because you don't feel worthy to receive, you are socially conditioned not to receive or have simply not practised receiving. Perhaps you were brought up to believe it is selfish to receive? Or it makes you needy? Or you will have to give more in payment than you receive and therefore you will lose out? None of these are true. It is one hundred percent OK to accept what is given and accept it with joy. It does not obligate you in any way.

Practise noticing the love and kindness and happiness the universe is offering you. Remember to actively look for what you are grateful for on a daily basis. By thanking the universe, you are telling it you are happy to receive more and more good things in your life. Be ready to accept the gifts you have asked the universe for in whatever way it wants to give them to you.

'Live in the faith that the whole world is on your side as long as you are true to the best that is in you.'

Christian D. Larson

MANIFESTING STORIES

PAIGE

'I saw my future partner in my imagination. I had a sense of his general height and colouring and a picture of us sitting together. In the picture, he made me laugh by telling me bad jokes. Five or so months later when I had given up on meeting him, I accepted an invitation to dinner with some friends. I sat next to a man I barely noticed until he started telling me jokes. You can guess the rest.'

FRANCESCA

'I thanked the universe in advance for doubling my income next year. I didn't need to write it down because it was so clear in my mind that it was possible for me to do so. I went through the year and did my accounts at the year end. I had earned exactly the amount I had imagined right down to the last penny.'

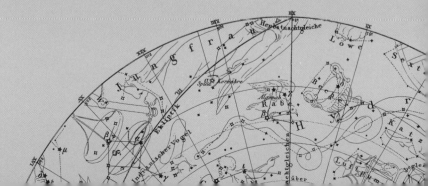

PETRA

'I asked the universe for a home and I imagined myself living there. I got a call a month later from a friend who wanted me to house sit for a year. I didn't own the home but it was exactly how I imagined it right down to the bath taps I had seen in a magazine. It was great but next time I manifested I made sure to imagine owning the home.'

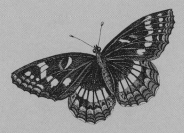

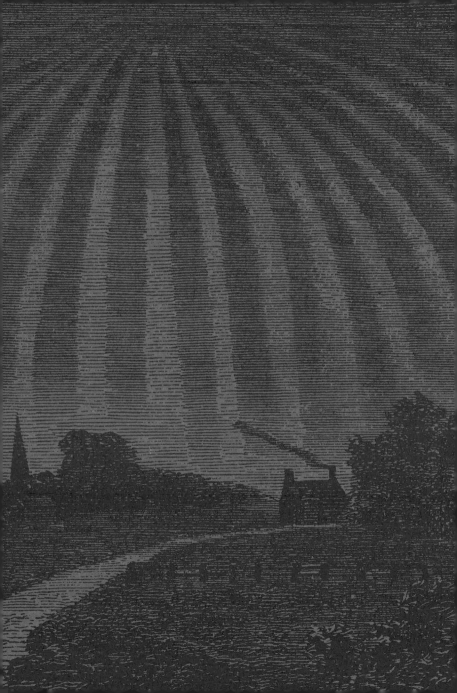

'Weak people talk and do not act, strong people act and keep silent.'

Éliphas Lévi

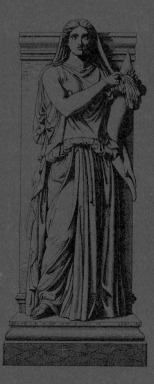

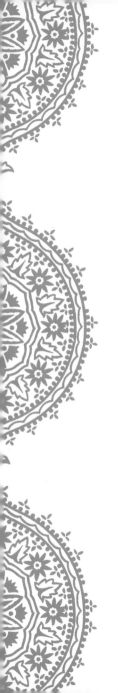

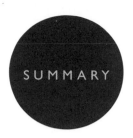

SUMMARY

COMMIT
and
TAKE ACTION
every day in the certainty
of manifesting.

✻

Practise THANK YOUs
every day.

✻

Replace scarcity thinking
with ABUNDANCE
thinking.

✻

Be ready to ACCEPT the
bountiful gifts of the universe
in whatever way the universe
presents them to you.

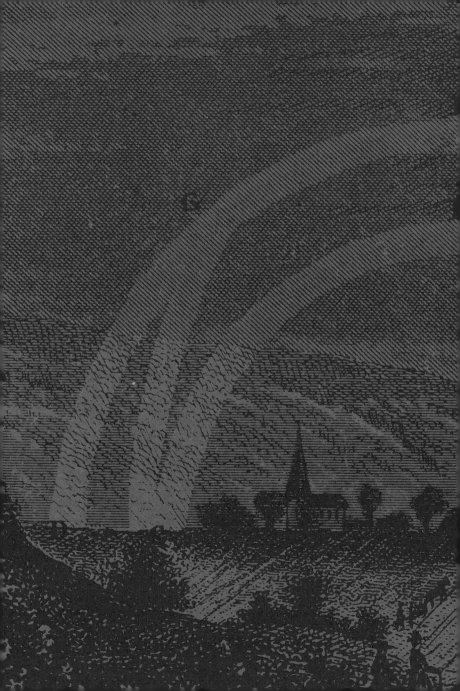

CHAPTER SIX

THE POWER

of

BELIEF

'Believe in yourself and all that you are. Know that there is something inside you that is greater than any obstacle.'

Christian D. Larson

I've seen *The Wizard of Oz* at least twenty times and the part which always made an impression on me when I was young was when the wizard granted the tin man, the cowardly lion and the scarecrow their wishes. The scarecrow wanted a brain, the lion wanted courage and the tin man wanted a heart. The wizard gave each of them something which would make them think he was giving them the gift they most desired. Then each of them found what they were looking for: the lion was no longer afraid; the tin man was able to feel love and the scarecrow was wise. Of course, the wizard was a conman. These abilities were already inside them, they just needed to believe they were there. The power of belief was so strong it worked.

Belief – The self-fulfilling prophecy

Beliefs are not superficial things. Even when you are doing everything else right, a limiting belief can block your success or an enabling belief can catapult you forward and bring you even more than you ever thought you could achieve.

Your life as it is today, is a total and accurate reflection of your inner world. Your feelings come from the beliefs you hold. To attract more positive experiences in the external world, you must begin with the interior world.

If you hold beliefs that the world is fearful,
you will attract more fear.

If you believe the world is bad you will
only attract more bad things.

If you believe the world is loving and you
deserve love you will attract love.

If you believe the world is abundant you will
manifest abundantly.

Your beliefs become a self-fulfilling prophecy. The universe is built by your imagination so you can change your universe today in this very moment if you truly believe and feel you can.

Beliefs are often deeply held and unconscious. We can develop our beliefs because of early life experiences or from the power of groupthink. Cultural, inherited

family and peer beliefs exert a strong influence on what we manifest.

It does take a lot of intention to step away from the crowd and truly believe something different. This is why it is so important to train your mind through imagination, visualisation and looking for evidence that you are successfully manifesting by building your manifests step by step.

As you are learning to manifest, step away from group think: turn off bad news, stop watching the media or scrolling through negative social media. Group thinking can be very powerful. Here's an example: if you look back at old films, forty-year-olds looked old. Now one-hundred-year-olds run marathons – as our group beliefs about age have changed so has how we look and feel at different ages.

Instead, find people with positive beliefs and adopt what they think about the world. Think about someone you really admire – I always choose Beyoncé when I am thinking about motivating beliefs because she seems to fit so much into her day! What do you think the person you've chosen believes about life?

'Nothing ever goes
away until it has
taught us what
we need to know.'

Pema Chödrön

'The pathway is smooth, why do you throw rocks before you?'

Ancient saying

THE LAW OF CAUSE AND EFFECT

The Law of Cause and Effect is a spiritual law which says that all actions you take will have a corresponding result exactly in proportion to it. To change your results, change your actions. If you keep on doing the same thing it will produce the same result.

Think about the actions you take and how they are taking you to your desired outcome. What is the likely effect of what you are doing now? What new actions could you take? Now, think about the physical environment you are building in your home. How does your physical environment affect and reflect your feelings and vice versa? What can you change in your physical environment to symbolise and confirm your commitment to manifest your desired outcome?

THE LAW OF POLARITY

The Law of Polarity is the principle that when energy manifests in our material world and takes form, it divides into pairs. This means that everything has an opposite or pole: love and hate, good and bad, hot and cold, fast and slow, loud and quiet, masculine and feminine. Think about the earth itself: it has a north and a south pole.

To get rid of something you don't like in your current world you need to think about the limiting belief and thoughts you hold which have given rise to it, then think about the polar opposite: what are the thoughts you want to hold instead? Then act in accordance with the new beliefs you wish to hold.

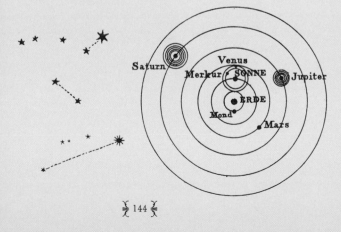

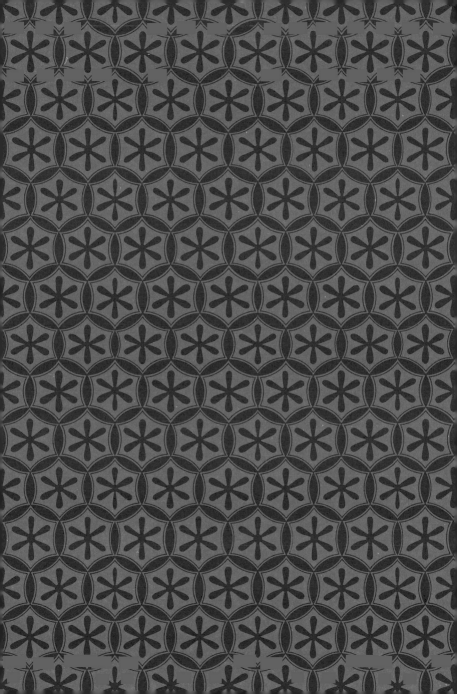

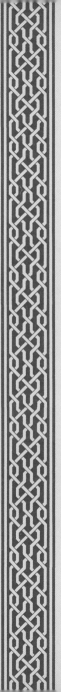

LIMITING BELIEFS

Have you ever noticed recurring patterns in your life? Attracting the same circumstance again and again? Attracting the same relationship with each partner? The same money patterns, the same cycles of feelings?

Patterns are a natural part of the universe. Think about the way we see patterns in nature: in the weather, or in the movements of flocks of birds. The universe loves patterns.

Mental patterns are a natural part of our complex inner worlds. They are a way our subconscious groups and processes important beliefs. These beliefs cause our behaviour and on a vibrational level cause what we attract and manifest.

When you notice a negative pattern in your life, spend some time thinking about what deep limiting beliefs you have about yourself and the world which underlie these patterns.

If you can interrupt a destructive or challenging pattern in your life you will create miraculous and positive change.

When I first started working with clients, I noticed how some people would come in with very fixed ideas about life. For example, a woman who had been cheated on told me, 'All men I meet cheat.' A man I worked with who was constantly rejected by women told me with great certainty, 'Women just don't commit nowadays.'

These statements may seem untrue to you and me but they were perfectly true to these two people because this is what they attracted in their lives. They vibrated these beliefs out to the universe and in return the universe obliged them by sending them more evidence to support these beliefs.

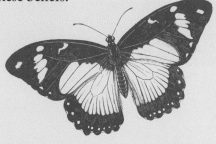

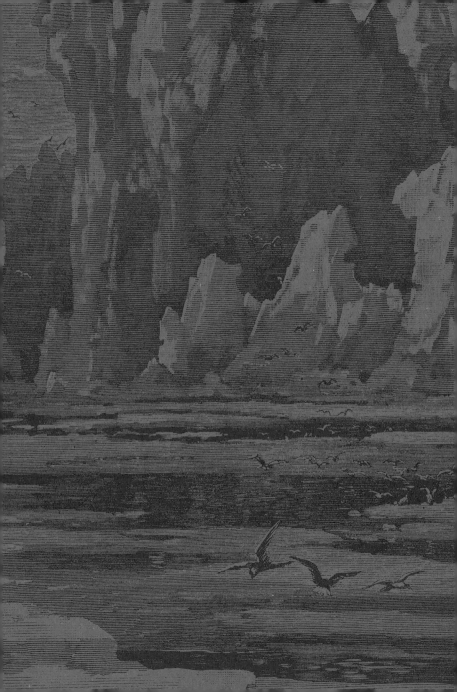

UNCOVERING YOUR BELIEFS

How do you know what you truly believe about the world? Look around you at what you have created. The life you have is the one you believe you can create. Change your beliefs and you will change the material world you live in. When you truly believe something to be true it will become true.

It is important to know what your beliefs about manifesting are. What do you think you have intentionally manifested in your life so far? Do you have an awareness of having visualised something happening in your future and having it come true? By searching for evidence to show that you have intentionally manifested in the past it will build your belief that you can do so in the future.

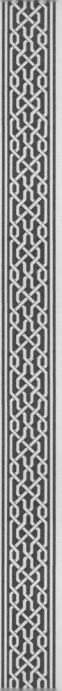

LIMITING BELIEFS

Sit quietly and think about an obstacle you have faced in the past.

✺ What limiting belief (s) do you have that attracted that obstacle to you?

✺ What is the polar opposite of this (these) belief (s)?

✺ Where are you feeling stuck in your life and what beliefs underlie this stuckness?

✺ What are your biggest fears and what beliefs underlie these fears?

✺ What do you feel you are incapable of changing and what beliefs underlie these feelings?

✺ What won't you change for fear of being judged and what beliefs underlie these fears?

※ What are you most resistant to and what beliefs underlie this resistance?

※ How do you limit the choices and opportunities in your life and what beliefs underlie this limiting?

※ What do you feel it is too late or too early to change and what beliefs underlie these feelings?

※ Who do you think you are and are not?

※ 'I am...'

※ 'I can...'

※ 'I am not...'

※ I can not...'

Now think about all the beliefs you want to hold instead.

CHANGING YOUR BELIEFS

Here's a simple way to change your beliefs. Become an evidence seeker.

Decide on a belief which you wish to hold instead of a previous limiting belief.

Now look for evidence to prove the new belief you want to hold as true. By actively searching out evidence to prove your new belief it will shift you towards genuinely holding the new belief. You will know how successfully you are doing this by the new experiences, thoughts, feelings, people and things you begin to manifest into your life.

If you are still not achieving success in manifesting, then you either haven't identified the key beliefs or haven't convinced your subconscious of the new beliefs.

Make sure you examine your beliefs about giving and receiving. Check to see if it is OK for you to receive unconditionally from the universe.

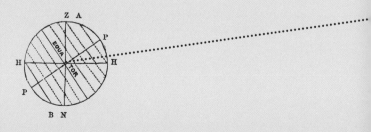

'The world is full
of obvious facts
which nobody by
any chance ever
observes.'

Arthur Conan Doyle

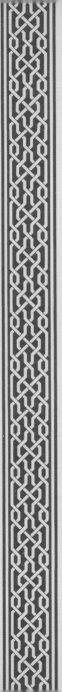

CHANGE YOUR LANGUAGE

The second way to change your beliefs is to challenge how you speak to yourself.

Listen to how you speak to yourself. Negative words are clues to negative subconscious beliefs. If you are carrying around negative beliefs, it's like dragging around a big black bag of low vibration in your subconscious which will disrupt your ability to manifest what you want.

Do you use the word 'everyone' in sentences, like: *'Everyone ends up lonely.'* That's a generalisation, not a fact.

Do you say things like, *'It's difficult for people like me to manifest.'* That's a limiting belief.

Do you say things like, *'I had one bad experience so that means things will go wrong forever.'* That's called catastrophising, where you expect the worst possible outcome.

Your life contains a lifetime of learning. The

words you choose to you speak to yourself and the beliefs that underlie these words have come about as a result of a lifetime of learning ways of thinking.

It is time to unlearn those which don't work.

If you hear yourself talking in negative generalisations and using words like, 'everyone' or 'always', stop and say to yourself:

'Everyone? Always? What if this *wasn't* true? Are there exceptions? What could I think instead which would be more empowering?'

If you hear yourself expressing a limiting belief, stop and ask yourself:

'What would an empowering belief be instead?'

If you hear yourself catastrophising, stop and ask yourself, 'What if I got a positive result this time?' Maybe, this time think, 'I had a bad experience and now things will go really well in future because I am thinking differently and attracting new energy in my life.'

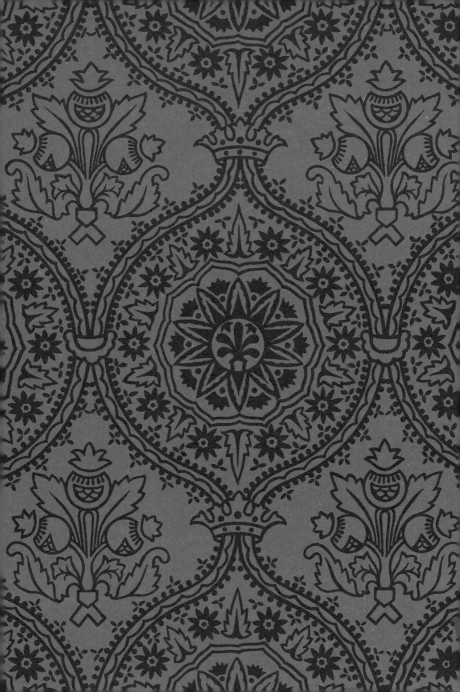

BELIEVE YOU ARE LUCKY

Research on luck has discovered that lucky people really do exist. They have good relationships, make money, enjoy their careers and have good jobs. It is nothing to do with their talents but everything to do with belief. Sometimes their belief comes because they were told when they were children they were lucky. Or the particular circumstances they experienced when young led them to just believe they were lucky.

These beliefs build luck. They lead people to be open to live life in a relaxed manner, assuming their future will work out well. This optimism brings in positive people and life experiences.

In other words, they are subconsciously manifesting positive things by vibrating this positive belief to the universe.

Believing you are lucky is one of the top beliefs which can change your world.

It is easy to adopt this belief.

The belief you want to prove is that you are a lucky person.

Now if you don't think you are I bet you can come

up with tons of evidence showing the bad luck in your life.

Changing this belief is just a matter of finding the opposite evidence. Here's how to do it.

Think about a time when things went well for you.

How did you feel in that moment?

Close your eyes and really get in touch with the feeling.

Next, deliberately ramp up this feeling so it

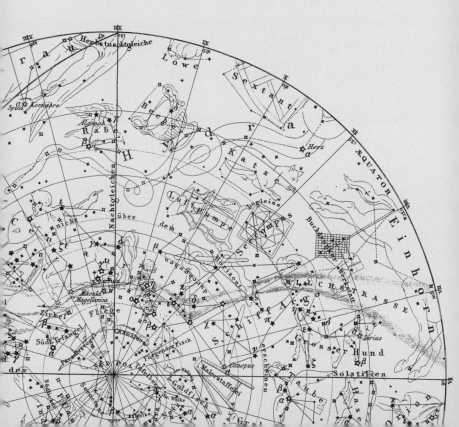

reverberates through your whole body.

Imagine your future in front of you like a line of time.

Visualise this wonderful feeling running into your future, filling up your timeline with luck and good experiences.

Open your eyes, take a breath and feel the positive feelings still in your body.

Now repeat this with another time when things went well for you.

I want you to make sure you repeat this at least one more time so you have a minimum of three experiences to draw on.

Finally say to yourself, 'I am a lucky person. *I am a very lucky person.*'

As you say this, let positive feelings fill your body and visualise yourself travelling into the future again pulling all the luck along with you and noticing the new life you are manifesting filled with exciting and happy experiences.

'No man ever steps
in the same river
twice, for it's not
the same river
and he's not the
same man.'

Heraclitus

CHANGING BELIEFS THROUGH SYMBOLS

Take any physical material such as clay or paper or plasticine. Make an image of a belief you don't want to hold. It can be an abstract image. As you make it, imagine putting any thoughts relating to this belief and any obstacles you have faced into the image you are making. You may find this a very meditative experience.

When you finish, immediately destroy what you have made. Crush it, burn it, pound it into pieces. Throw it away.

Then straight away take some fresh material and construct an image which represents what you are now going to manifest in your life. As you make this think about the new beliefs you are right now taking on which support you manifesting this in your life.

Keep this image somewhere you can look at it or notice it as you go about your daily life and it will become a prompt for your subconscious to get going on manifesting your desired outcome and changing your life.

Make any appropriate adjustments to the image so it continues to inspire you.

MANIFESTING STORY

JULIE

Julie was adopted when she was young and had always suffered from feelings of inadequacy. Even when she made money and entered into a relationship she repeatedly seemed to subconsciously sabotage her life so that she lost the money and the relationship failed. What she seemed to want subconsciously was to prove again and again that she would be loved for herself regardless of whether she had money. She worked out a clear picture of what she desired to manifest and made sure she got the positive feelings associated with what she wanted.

Simultaneously, she spent a considerable amount of time writing down all the limiting beliefs she had around money, relationships and love. She stepped tentatively into a new relationship and as past feelings came up she made sure she identified the beliefs underlying them and focused again and again on what she wanted, not the patterns she had previously created. So far she is successfully several years into a relationship and her wealth is growing.

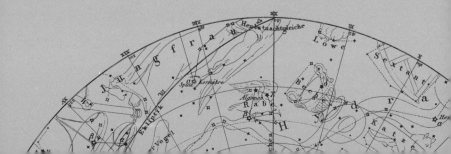

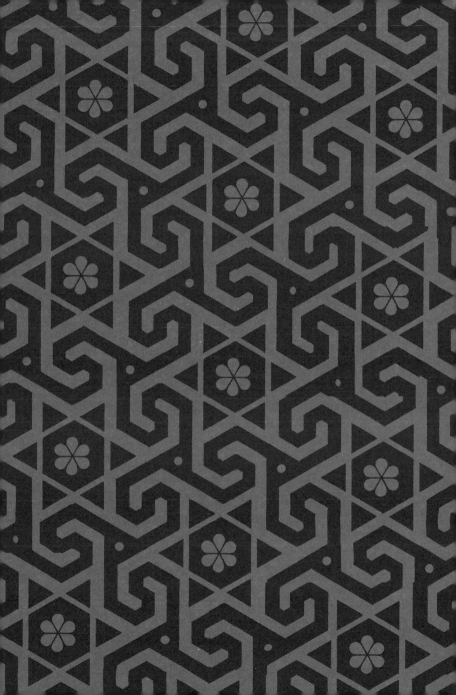

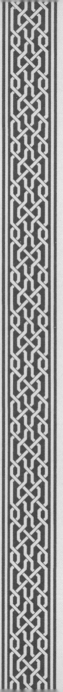

MANIFESTING MONEY

A lot of people have blocking beliefs around making money especially when they came from a power background full of scarcity beliefs.

Money is only energy like everything else. If you know you have blocking beliefs around money, start small.

You will manifest money most effectively if you link it to a material desire you wish to pay for. In this way you create a need the universe will recognise. Imagine a small thing you would like to buy. Now imagine the money coming to you easily and from a source which makes you feel good. I'm not talking millions here but a few notes. When people do this exercise, they tell me they visualise paying for what they want, finding money they had lost in their purse, a friend repaying a loan, finding money in the street or even getting a small win on the lottery. The universe has infinite ways of getting manifests to you.

Practise this exercise so you get comfortable manifesting small amounts.

Now use some of the ideas below to create a feeling of flow and abundance.

Every time you get a bill, say thank you. Open those credit card statement with joy and thank the universe for providing you with the means to pay them.

Write yourself a cheque for the amount of money you need for something you want to manifest in your life. Stick the cheque on a vision board, or the mirror where you look at yourself every morning or somewhere else.

Do you invoice a client regularly or receive a pay cheque from an employer? Print off a copy and change the amount of money to the amount you need for your next big manifest.

Gratefully, pay for gifts for others knowing that you will receive the same amount or more back in one form or another from the universe.

When you receive money from the universe say thank you and appreciate the gift you have received.

As you build up a trail of evidence that you can manifest, you will overcome any negative scarcity beliefs.

'It is good to love many things, for therein lies strength, and whosoever loves much performs much, and can accomplish much, and what is done with love is well done.'

Vincent van Gogh

THE LAW OF COMPENSATION

According to this spiritual law you will receive back in life exactly what you put in. It is another way of expressing the idea that you reap what you sow. It is similar to the Law of Attraction but the difference is to express that you will receive back exactly what you put into life big and small. It is a reminder to us that we get back what we deserve.

If you treat the whole world well, you will receive good things in return. If you send out love you will receive compensation.

For example, if you desire to manifest riches but treat the world badly along the way, you may get the riches you want but become unhappy with the effect of them.

When you state the desire you want to manifest, make sure you add a statement like this:

'Thank you for now manifesting xxx as long as it is good for me, others around me and the world as a whole.'

Remember, absolutely everything in our universe is interconnected. You can't NOT affect other people and the world as a whole with every action, thought, desire and manifest you have.

The only way to have a positive effect is always to act with a positive and loving intention. Check your feelings. Make sure you manifest with pure love in your heart.

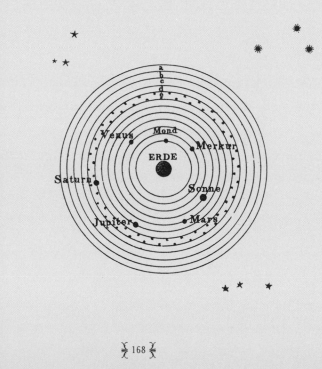

'All the earth is mine, and I have a right to go all over it and through it.'

Apollonius of Tyana

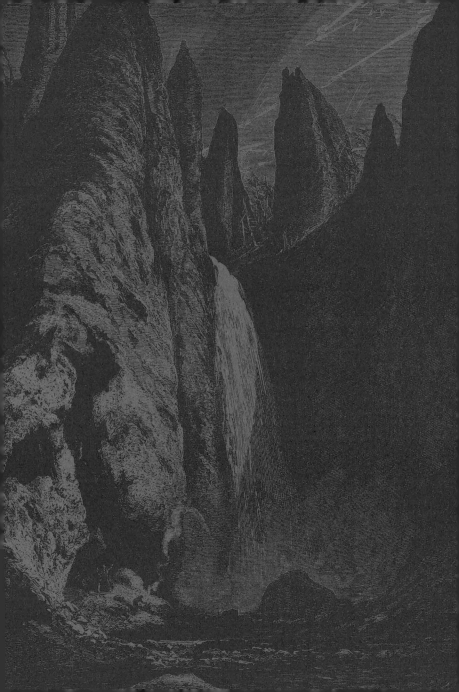

THE LAW OF PERPETUAL TRANSMUTATION

This spiritual law reminds us is that the universe is made of energy so it is impossible for it not to change. As part of this universe, you are also constantly changing.

As energy moves between the spiritual and physical worlds it brings things into being and dissolves them again. We live and die. So does every physical thing in the universe. Your physical body for example may look as if it is solid but in fact every cell and organ is constantly rebuilding itself.

The energy of the life force does not die. It is timeless and without end. It cannot be destroyed. It simply transmutes from the spiritual universe where things are formless into matter and a particular form, then out of matter back to spirit and then into matter again in a new form. This cycle of transmutation continues forever.

Your life is the same. It cannot stay still. This means that you can change anything in your life at any point.

'All that we are is the result of what we have thought: it is founded on our thoughts and made up of our thoughts. If a man speaks or acts with an evil thought, suffering follows him as the wheel follows the hoof of the beast that draws the wagon... If a man speaks or acts with a good thought, happiness follows him like a shadow that never leaves him.'

Buddha

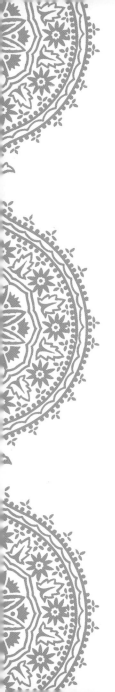

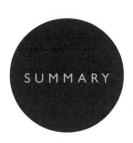

SUMMARY

Your BELIEFS can
limit or empower you.

※

Become aware of your deep-held
beliefs through examining the
results you get in your life.

※

It's OK to separate yourself from
group beliefs and be different.

※

Look for people who have success
in areas you want to emulate
and adopt their beliefs.

※

CHANGE your limiting beliefs to
EMPOWERING BELIEFS.

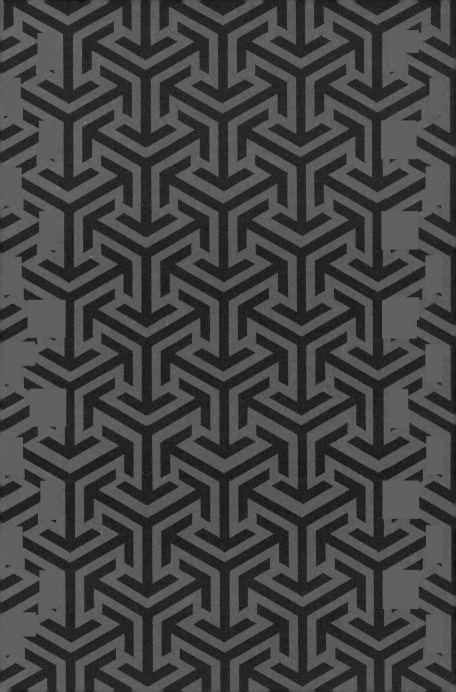

CHAPTER SEVEN

HABIT

'We are what we repeatedly do. Excellence, then, is not an act, but a habit.'

Will Durant

Your habits are what define you. Your life is the creation of every thought and habit you have. Every habit determines your day ahead and each day determines what life you lead. Since manifesting always takes the path of least resistance, to change your life you need to build new habits of thinking and action into your life which support your aims and intentions.

We become loving by being loving, brave by taking brave actions, happy by focusing on happy thoughts and experiences. Think about changing your life in small steps day by day, week by week, month by month and you will soon find big changes manifesting.

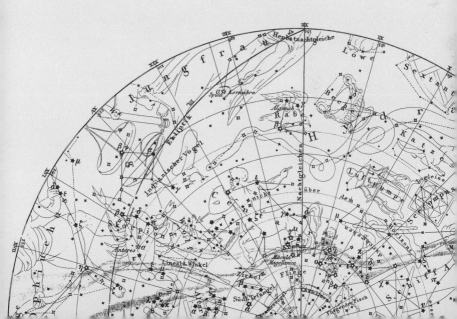

'Every morning we are born again. What we do today is what matters most.'

Buddha

SPIRITUAL LAW 12
THE LAW OF ACTION

It is not enough to want something or visualise it. You must align your action to what you want to manifest by taking active steps. This shows the universe you are serious and committed to that goal and will attract the job you want, the new life you want or the relationship you want.

It doesn't need to be a big step. A first step sets your intention and then as opportunities arrive you can take more steps and form new habits.

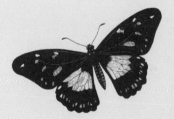

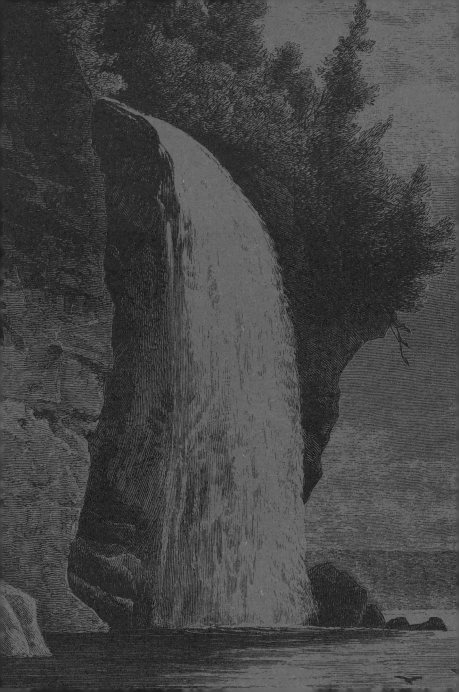

BUILD SUCCESS AWARENESS

Each day revisit your manifests and see how you feel about them. As a daily ritual: every morning, reflect on the statement of your desired outcome and say it to yourself to keep your thoughts fixed upon it. Give yourself time away from other people so you have space to really focus on what you are doing. Carve out pockets of silence in your day so you can get in touch with what you really want.

Pause also and recognise your successes. Think about something you have done well. It could be something you have made, or learned, or taught, or caused to happen.

Think about the sequence of events which led to this result.

How did you contribute positively to this?

What actions did you take however small which showed the universe your intention?

There is no limit to the impact you can have on your world, only the limit of your beliefs and commitment.

BUILD ORDER AND CONSISTENCY

Order helps to create successful manifesting. Create prompts to remind your subconscious every day about the life you desire to manifest. Here are some different prompts you can use.

※ Make an image of what you want. You can do this in different ways. Collect photographs from magazines and make a physical vision board of your ideal future or make a vitual vision board on your computer or phone.

※ Create a physical symbol using clay or another medium to represent what you desire to manifest. It's OK if it's abstract. It doesn't need to look like what you wish to manifest. It just has to have personal meaning for you.

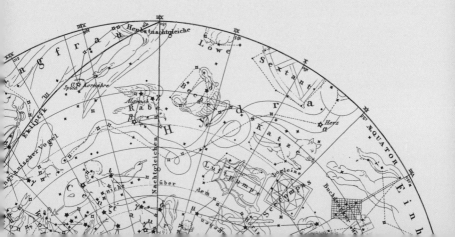

'Great things are done by a series of small things brought together.'

Vincent van Gogh

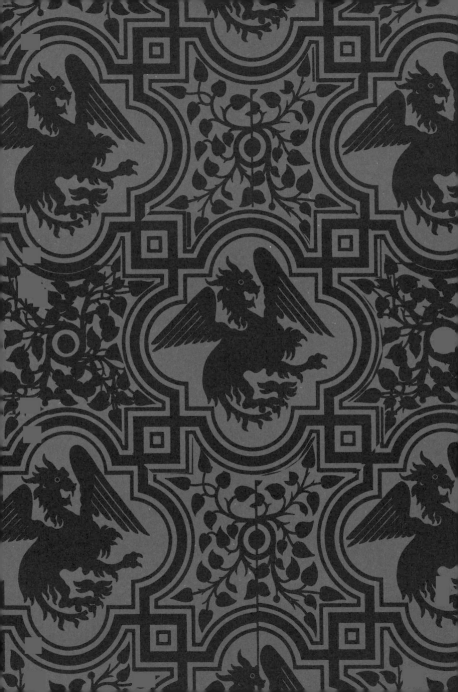

✺ Make yourself a personal altar. Take a private area in your home where others can't interfere with what you put there. It can even be in a cupboard drawer. Gather or collect objects which represent your manifesting intentions and place them on this altar.

✺ Let your mind go to these places and pictures and symbols often so you can check in to see if they are still the right representations for you.

YOUR PHYSICAL BODY

Here is a great morning ritual which will make you start the day feeling physically energised. The physical, emotional and spiritual bodies are all linked, so by doing this you will help yourself manifest successfully.

Look at yourself in the mirror. Even if you have suffered sickness or injury your body gives you so much.

The body is constantly repairing and renewing itself. Your subconscious mind has a blueprint from birth of what a perfectly functioning body is. Believe that you can renew and refresh every cell in your body and restore that blueprint to perfect health and wellbeing.

'Start a huge, foolish
project, like Noah…
it makes absolutely
no difference what
people think of you.'

Rumi

This morning ritual builds positive beliefs about your physical health, youth and wellbeing.

- ☀ Sit and look at yourself in a mirror. Take a few slow, deep breaths to still your mind. Let your spine be in a straight, upright position with your head balancing on a relaxed neck and shoulders.

- ☀ Look at your face and notice all the colours in your eyes.

- ☀ Notice your skin and the tiny differences in shades from your forehead to your nose, cheeks and chin.

- ☀ Notice your mouth. Think about how amazing it is that just by eating good food you send health to every part of your body.

- ☀ If you can see your whole body in the mirror, notice how amazing the human body truly is. It allows you to live in this incredible, complex physical world. Appreciate the material form you have now and thank the universe for the good health which is now flowing to you.

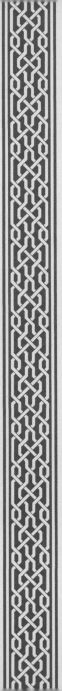

Now, build positive energy for the day

❀ Smile gently to yourself with the sides of your mouth tilting upwards gently. Allow your eyes to smile too. Now breathe out and let go.

❀ Flow the loving energy of this smile throughout your body. See that love flowing from the universe to your heart, your lungs, your spleen, your kidneys, your stomach, and your adrenal glands. Imagine, as the love flows to your inner organs it renews and restores them to perfect functioning. You can see them flooded with the loving energy of this smile, healing them and letting go of any emotional, physical and mental energies you don't want any more.

❀ Finish, by seeing the loving smile energy gather in your naval, energising you throughout the day to come.

'A path is made by walking on it.'

Zhuangzi

'Both success and
failure are largely
the results of habit.'

Napoleon Hill

ETHICAL MANIFESTING

As you build manifesting habits into your daily life, set a clear intention to act with integrity in everything you do. Sometimes people get impatient and try shortcuts to wealth or love but they won't bring you happiness. Only working with the loving universe will do that.

A word about free will. You cannot use manifesting and the Law of Attraction to overcome someone's free will to choose. This means you can't force someone to love you (which is one of the most frequently asked questions). They can't force you either.

You also have free will to do the wrong thing, therefore think very carefully about what you want to manifest and why.

Will it really get the result you want? There are countless fairytales around the world warning us about people who are given three wishes only to find that what they thought they wanted had unintended consequences for them.

Generally just wishing for wealth for yourself won't bring you happiness. Think about where true happiness lies in your life. In physical health? Family? Mental health? Leaving a positive legacy for the world?

THE MONKEY'S PAW
BE CAREFUL WHAT YOU WISH FOR

In the cautionary tale of *The Monkey's Paw* by W. W. Jacobs, published in 1902, Mr White is given a stuffed monkey's paw. He is told it will give him three wishes, but it is dangerous to use them because there is a curse attached: when the paw grants your wish there will be a price to pay.

Mr White asks for £200 to pay off his mortgage. The money comes to him but only as compensation for his son being fatally injured in an accident. His desperate wife asks him to wish their son alive again. This second wish is granted but they are terrified of the non-human who appears at the door to their home. Mr White uses his final wish to get rid of 'the thing outside' and the couple are left alone, with their mortgage paid but no son.

'The man who moves a mountain begins by carrying away small stones.'

Confucius

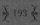

Here are some suggestions to bring positive habits into your life which will help your energy to stay high. High energy will magnetise good outcomes into your life.

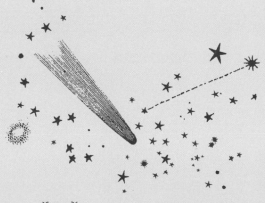

MONDAY

Today is about your home. Create outer order to help your inner order. In a clean, fresh space you know what exists in your life and you can create space to bring new things in. Each Monday, spend a little time spring cleaning and clearing old stuff out of your home: clothes and unwanted ornaments, etc. and start creating your home as near as you can to the vision you want. Bring in symbols of your new life and place them where you can see them. It's OK to throw stuff out because it's soon going to be replaced by new things. Get rid of broken and chipped objects. Look at everything you own and think, does this give me joy or is this genuinely useful in my life? If it is, keep it. After you spring clean, you may want to refresh the energy in your home by burning sage or aromatherapy oils, or simply opening the windows and letting fresh air come in. Why not bring flowers into your home as well? Think intentionally as you do this about bringing fresh energy into your home with each action you take.

P.S. If you are looking for a relationship remember to leave some space for your future partner to put their things.

TUESDAY

Today is about your emotional body. This is a day to remember to forgive. Sit quietly and think about the people you have encountered in your life. This includes family, friends and people who have passed through your life but are no longer with you. How do you see them in your mind's eye? Do you have feelings of joy about them or are your feelings more mixed? Imagine you have a stage in front of you and you can bring each person on stage so you can talk to them. Now have a conversation with love. Say what you need to say in a loving voice and listen to what they have to say in return. When this conversation is held in love, you will be able to forgive them for any hurt done to you and you will hear forgiveness from them. Now let them go and allow them to leave. You can repeat this for as many weeks as you like. Today is also a day to give freely. You are part of the abundant universe so by forgiving and giving freely you will create more abundance. Think about doing a small act of kindness for a neighbour, friend or stranger. Write a note to someone you have lost touch with. Pass on some of your good fortune by giving time or money to someone in need. Luck is simply another word for successful manifesting. Pass on some of your good luck.

WEDNESDAY

Remember that a healthy emotional body, a healthy physical body and a healthy mental body all feed each other. Today is the day to think about your physical body: the food you eat and the exercise you do. This doesn't mean rushing off to the gym, it could just mean putting on some music and dancing. Move your body and feel the life force of the universe bringing you good health. Open your fridge and look at what you are going to eat today. Does it look full of life force? When you walk into a store full of vibrant, coloured vegetables and fresh produce you can feel good energy coming from it. If you walk into the middle aisles of the supermarket where the highly packaged, ultra-processed food lives it appears full of dull energy. That's because it lacks life force.

THURSDAY

Today is the day to open your heart. Sit quietly and place both hands on your heart. As you breathe, consciously imagine opening up your heart centre as if the petals of a rose are unfolding. You can imagine a rose pink or white light filling this centre. Notice when you do this how in touch you feel with your loving self. If any thoughts or ideas come to you, do write them down afterwards. If you feel your heart is really blocked there is a release you can do. Turn on the taps and hold your hands under running water while rubbing them with salt. Salt is a great cleanser and will release any negative energies you have. If that is still not enough, take an Epsom salts bath and feel heavy energy lift away from your body.

FRIDAY

Know yourself and your truth. Often we hold back from communicating with others honestly and even communicating truthfully with ourselves. We have all had the experience of suppressing thoughts or emotions we don't want to have or we are afraid will have negative consequences. The throat is the centre of communication in the body. Imagine, as you breathe, opening up the centre of your throat, like the petals of a rose unfurling. Open your mouth and let out a deep breath and expel all those negative words and emotions you have held contained in your throat. Why not start this morning or finish the day by writing freely in a journal. Just write whatever comes to your mind about what you feel about yourself, the world or other people. This is only for you so there is no need to censor or judge yourself. It is simply an exercise to free yourself up. In fact, after you have written whatever you want to write, you don't need to look at it again. You can scrunch it up and throw it away.

SATURDAY

Today is your grounding day. If you want to connect more with nature, walk barefoot in the garden, sit in silence in the natural world and take time to connect to the earth. As you walk or sit, imagine you have roots growing out of your feet and going deep into the earth. You are now grounded in the earthy world. When you feel grounded, imagine the top of your head opening up and letting in the light of the universe. Your body is now a pure channel for the life force from the highest frequencies of the universe to connect to matter.

SUNDAY

Today is the day you will rest well. Set aside time for silence or meditation. Turn off your electronic devices several hours before you sleep. Let your body find its natural sleep rhythm by going to sleep when you feel tired. Dull your lights when the sun goes down and see if you can rise when the sun rises each morning. If you wake up with the sun, you connect with the natural cycles of the universe. This rhythm helps you to connect with nature as well as every living creature and part of the material world and, ultimately, more deeply with yourself.

Every day remember to be grateful and remember all the good things which have happened for you and thank the universe again for the abundance it brings.

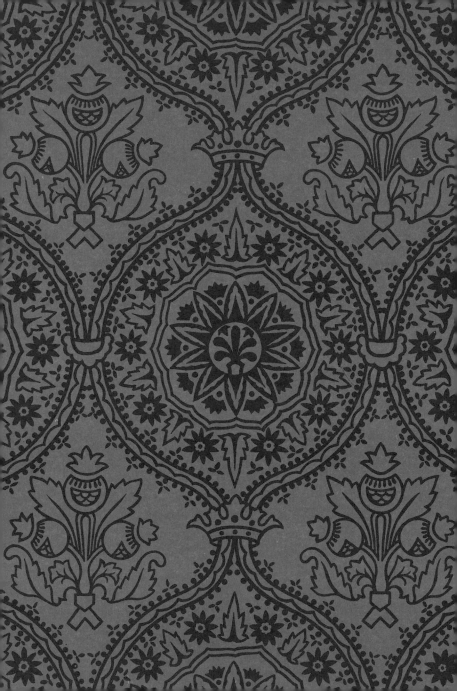

'Don't wait. The time will never be just right.'

Napoleon Hill

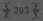

'To leave the
world richer –
that is the
ultimate success.'

Eleanor Roosevelt

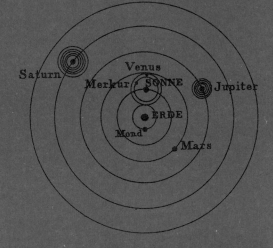

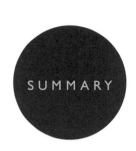

SUMMARY

HABITS instil order and consistency of
thought, feelings and actions.
Through new habit forming you will
bring your mental, emotional, spiritual
and physical bodies into good shape
and align them with what you
desire to manifest.

❋

Use the seven days in your week wisely.
You can use the habit prompts
in the book or come up with your
own routines.

❋

Through habit you can overcome
thinking blocks and bring miracles
into your life.

❋

Through building new habits you will
make the Law of Attraction work most
powerfully for you.

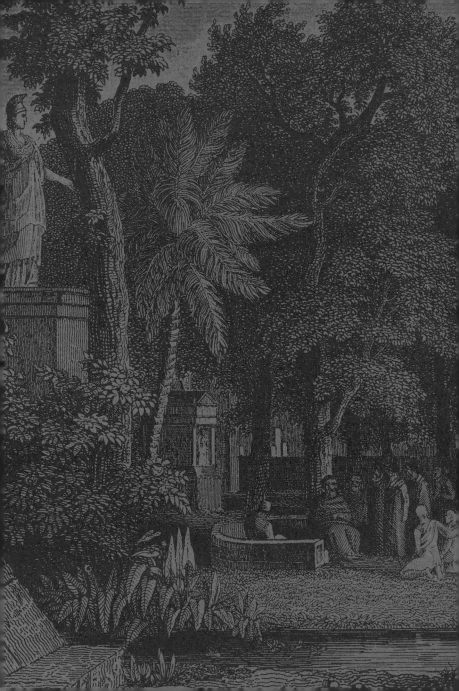

CHAPTER EIGHT

MANIFEST

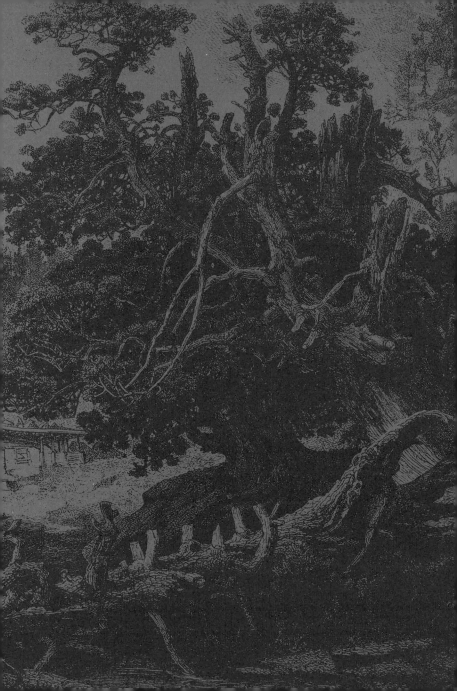

'A man's mind may be likened to a garden, which may be intelligently cultivated or allowed to run wild; but whether cultivated or neglected, it must, and will, bring forth. If no useful seeds are put into it, then an abundance of useless weed seeds will fall therein, and will continue to produce their kind.'

James Allen

This chapter is written for your subconscious not your conscious mind. It contains a guided visualisation just for you. Everyone's experience is different and each time you do this it may be different. That's perfect and how it is supposed to be. Simply pick a time when you can be alone and find quiet. You can either sit straight backed in a chair or lie down. Rest your arms and hands in a comfortable position. Make sure your body is comfortable and supported.

Relax.

Close your eyes.

Take a deep breath... hold it ... let it out all the way... and another breath ... and this time really relax and you let the breath all the way out.

And one more breath and allow your whole body to relax ...

Be aware of the weight of your arms and legs as they go heavy ... and you go deeper ... and your whole body is so comfortable.

Remember when you were a child what it was like to open a book full of pictures and find yourself in new worlds full of magic and wonder. Imagine you are opening the first page and there in front of you is a door to a magic world.

You can reach out to the handle of the door and turn it and step through the open door now.

You find yourself in a garden on a hot, sunny day. The temperature is pleasantly warm and inviting. Here in front of you is an armchair in the middle of the grass surrounded by flowers and trees. Imagine now settling down in the chair feeling so comfortable knowing this is a place you can look around in peace and security.

The garden is safe. It belongs to you and only you can determine what you have in this garden.

The garden is silent apart from a strange feeling, I wonder if you can feel it ... the anticipation of some magical and wonderful event.

You find yourself noticing the beautiful flowers and more trees and long grass and paths winding into the distance. You are aware of the pleasant perfumes of flowers filling the air.

You are filled with curiosity to find out more about the garden. You get up from the armchair and begin to walk through the long grass and along one of the many paths. As you do so, you notice the sounds of bees and insects flitting around the blossoms and birds flying overhead and calling from the tall trees.

You walk on, not really sure of where you are going until in the distance you catch sight of a gold light. You are filled with desire to see what lies within the gold light so you walk through the garden following the most direct path you can following the gold light.

At the end of the garden a light mist begins to gather, swirling around you and obscuring the way. But if you keep walking as the mist twists and turns around

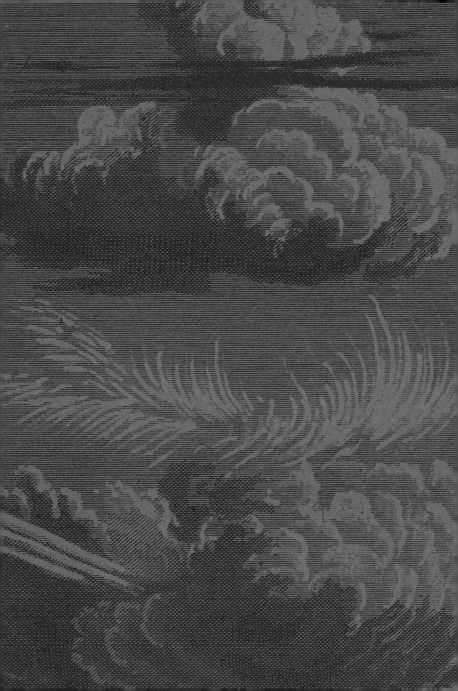

you, you are certain the way will become clear.

The mist is sparkling and light. With every step forward you take, time seems to shift and still. Your breathing is deeper now, softer and comfortable. You are drifting, carried forward by the mist.

As the mists begin to settle down, you see there is a rocky path ahead and then a murky swamp. Nevertheless, the thought of the gold light carries you forward and you find as you walk, your feet find a steady foothold despite the seemingly hard conditions.

There are distractions along the way: you have glimpses of other side paths you can take, and at times you wonder whether it might be less effort to go back to the garden and forget the journey. But then the gold light reappears and somehow you keep going.

Soon you find the rocky path and swamp have gone. You are on solid ground again. You have hints of green again under your feet and you hear water in the distance. The path winds round through the remaining mist until from somewhere in the distance you see the mists lift to reveal what looks like a vast pool of water filling all the space up to the horizon.

As you approach, you notice the water. It is many shades of turquoise and blue and at some points obsidian black. You notice too that the water is shallow on the edge but little eddies and ripples reveal deeper places. You look up and notice that the sky is also a pool of rich sparkling blue which touches the water so softly but so securely there is no way to separate the two. In fact, the more you look at both, it is hard to tell which is which.

You step closer until you are standing by the edge of the pool.

The gold light is now above and inside the pool.

Lean forward and touch the water. See the ripples spread across the water.

The water is as opaque as a mirror.

As you look into the pool the ripples change to show glimpses of pictures from your life, people and events and sounds and feelings.

You understand somehow the pool is offering you the chance to revisit any event and see it from a new viewpoint and experience it in a fresh way…whatever way you choose to … and change the feelings … you have the opportunity to rewrite your past and write your future. It is all in the gift of the pool.

The waters change again and you see the future changing in front of you and you realise the future is still being written. It is not yet fixed. You can imagine the future how you want it to be and that will be so.

In fact, as you imagine a beautiful event in your future you see the picture appearing in the pool in front of you.

Stay here as long as you like and when you are ready, open your eyes and remember your future exactly as you want it to be.

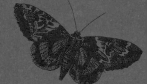

'There is
sunshine after
every rainfall.'

German proverb

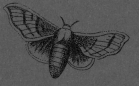

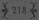

THANK YOU

Finally, I want to say *thank you* to you for reading *The Art of Manifesting*. As I said right at the beginning, we are all interconnected so just by reading this book you are helping me and others, create an even more wonderful universe and life experience.

You are in the perfect moment right now, a perfect person created by the life force. Have faith now as you continue along on the journey of life that if there are any swamps or rocky parts of the journey or times when it is so misty you can't see what is ahead of you, that you will reach that golden light and the next time you take a path it will become straighter and simpler.

You can manifest. You can change. You can create the life you want.

I wish you joy and love and success in manifesting the life of your dreams that helps to build a wonderful world for you and all of us.

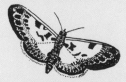

SUMMARY

The world is as you think it is.
To change your world, change
your thoughts.

ꙮ AWAKEN ꙮ

Love and happiness are yours by
right. Let go of pain and suffering.
The time to live as you want to live
is right now. Don't wait. There will
never be a better time.

ꙮ RECOGNISE YOUR POWER ꙮ

All power comes from within you
because you share the same power as
the whole universe. You are a centre
of expression for the life force which
creates and sustains everything in
existence. You have all the tools you
will ever need to begin.

⤙ ASK ⤚

Determine what you desire using
your free will. There are no limits.
Anything is possible. You can always
draw on the limitless richness the
universe supplies. Check what you
desire is good for you and the world.

⤙ IMAGINE ⤚

A weak desire will attract weak
results, but a well-formed desire
and focus will be rewarded. Use
the power of your subconscious
to imagine vividly what you want,
experiencing the joy you will feel
when your desire is fulfilled.

⤙ BELIEVE ⤚

Check your beliefs are aligned
with your desires. Believe before
you see the evidence.

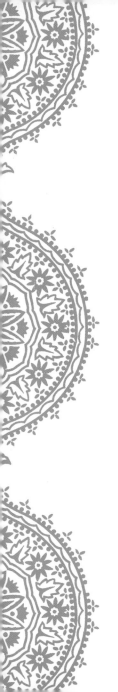

❧ LET GO ❧

Now let go of overattachment
to what you want to manifest.

❧ ACT ❧

Take actions towards your
future life in the confidence
what you desire will manifest.

❧ RECEIVE ❧

Practise receiving with
gratitude and build the world
you want to live in.

❧ MANIFEST ❧

Again and again until you
truly believe the evidence of
your own eyes.

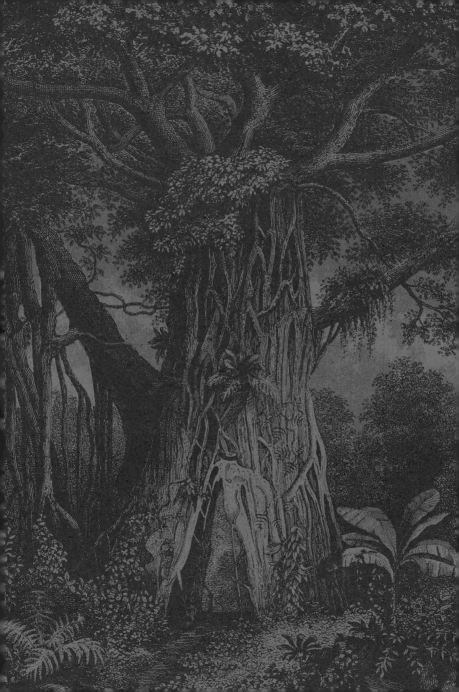

'The purpose of life is to live it, to taste experience to the utmost, to reach out eagerly and without fear for newer and richer experience.'

Eleanor Roosevelt

NOTES

NOTES

NOTES

NOTES

_____

_____

_____

_____

_____

_____

_____

_____

_____

_____

_____

_____

_____

_____

_____

NOTES

NOTES

NOTES

NOTES

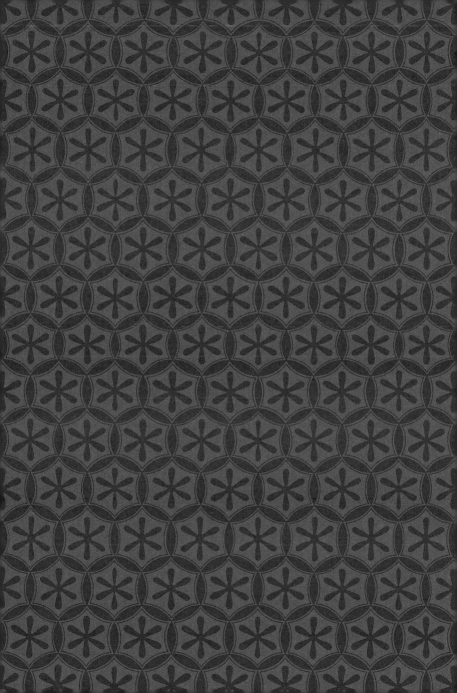

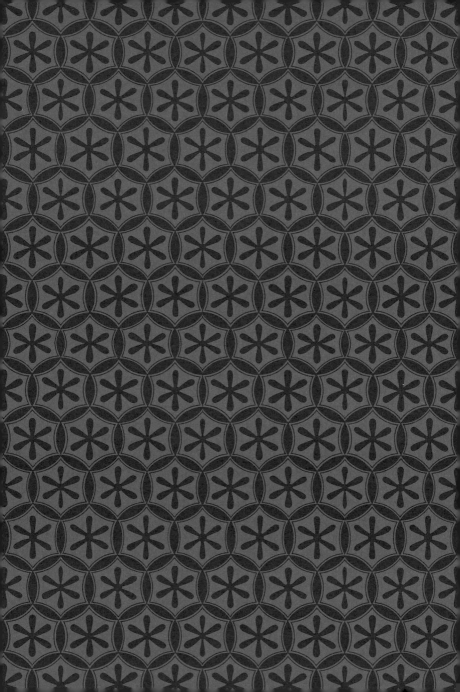